Interm

Fasting for

Women

The Ultimate Guide to How You Can Use This Science to Support Your Hormones, Weight Loss and Live a Healthy Life. How to Combine the 16/8 Method with Keto Diet

Additionally, the information in the following pages is intended only for informational purposes and should thus be thought of as universal. As befitting its nature, it is presented without assurance regarding its prolonged validity or interim quality. Trademarks

that are mentioned are done without written consent and can in no way be considered an endorsement from the trademark holder.

Table of Contents

Introduction

Congratulations on purchasing this book, and thank you for doing so. This book has been specifically designed for women who want to get the full advantage of intermittent fasting for weight loss and other health benefits.

Intermittent fasting has emerged as the new craze of the time. The reasons are obvious; it is highly effective and brings results. However, to get the best results, it is important that you understand the process completely and don't miss out on the intricate and important details.

Intermittent fasting is a great way to lose weight and burn fat. However, the advantages of intermittent fasting are not limited to that. It is also a way to attain holistic health improvement. Following an intermittent fasting routine in a proper way can bring an improvement in your overall health biomarkers too. But, at the same time, if you don't follow the routine properly or overdo some things, there can be side-effects, especially for women.

The purpose of this book is to explain intermittent fasting from the perspective of women. It is specifically aimed at women because incorrect fasting can have a devastating impact on the physical and mental health of women.

This book will just not give you the ways to lose weight with the help of intermittent fasting but also explain in detail the ways in which you can move towards better health. It will explain the main reasons behind the piling up of fat deposits and the ways our lifestyle is responsible for it.

Intermittent fasting is simply a moderation of the lifestyle to get out of the vicious cycle of weight gain and chronic health disorders.

This book will explain the complete processes and well as the reasons for doing things in the specific ways they are advised. It will give you a thorough understanding of the whole process of intermittent fasting.

It would also explain the concept of a Ketogenic diet or the keto diet and how it can accentuate the health benefits when coupled with intermittent fasting.

You will be able to understand the principles of the keto diet and the science behind it. You would also get a better understanding of your caloric requirements as well as the food basics.

This book will also help you in understanding the ways to make both these principles work together.

Most people get over-enthusiastic while telling about any new routine, and they also don't want to bring negative things into perspective. However, this can be very dangerous for the user. This book will also explain the side effects you can face while practicing intermittent fasting and the things you must always keep in mind while following the routine.

This book is a sincere attempt to help you understand the principles of intermittent fasting and the ways it can help you not only in losing weight but also in gaining better health. In this book, nothing has been sugar-coated to make things look rosier than they actually are. I've tried my best to keep the facts in front of you and cut the clutter so that you can have a better understanding of the concept for clear judgment.

I hope that you will be able to get the full advantage of this book.

There are plenty of books on this subject on the market, thanks again for choosing this one! Every effort was made to ensure it is full of as much useful information as possible; please enjoy it!

Chapter 1: Why Should We Worry?

An Overview of the Problem

Obesity is a condition we are not unfamiliar with. Whether we like it or not, it is there. Either you can try to get rid of it or learn to live with it. Most people feel the stress as they start gaining weight. In their desperation, they try every trick in the book.

However, there are exceptions too. There are people who remain chilled out.

- Some people might really find their love handles cute
- Some may even embrace oodles of fat with a smile
- Some carefree souls simply may not care about expanding physical frames
- Other courageous ones may even like carrying their chubby figures with pride

And all this is good, adorable, and admirable...............

Whatever way you take obesity, making a joke of it is not acceptable.

Fat shaming is bad. A person must never feel threatened, ashamed, humiliated, or anxious simply by virtue of possessing a different body type.

Doing that or being a cause of that in any manner is appalling, offensive, and criminal.

However, this doesn't mean overweight or obese women don't long for a frame that gives them more freedom and convenience.

It also doesn't undermine the fact that obesity is the leading cause of most of the preventable deaths in the modern world. It is a real problem that's staring at us right now in the form of an **Epidemic**. Irrespective of the fact that you feel comfortable in your skin or not, obesity is going to have a negative impact nonetheless.

The National Institute of Health (NIH) report states that obesity is the second leading cause of preventable deaths in the US. More than 300,000 people lose their lives here annually, a majority of them women. This is not even scratching the surface.

Even stating that obesity is a big problem is an **Understatement**.

- Obesity increases the risk of diabetes several times
    - **Did you know** that almost 80% of diabetic women are overweight or obese?
- Obesity escalates the risk of **PCOS**
    - **Did you know** that even a meager 5-7% reduction in weight can help in restoring the hormonal balance and bring relief in the symptoms of PCOS?
- Obesity increases the risk of heart diseases
    - **Did you know** that generally, 1 in 8 people die of heart diseases, but in women, this rate is 1 in 5? In obese and diabetic women, this risk further increases by 50% as compared to men with the same ailments.
- Obesity can affect your Mental Agility
    - A study conducted by researchers from Iowa State University has revealed that high belly fat leads to faster degradation of mental agility. Obesity

and related causes lead to a decrease in the mental agility of the victims.

Considering obesity, a mere cosmetic problem is one of the biggest mistakes you will make. It has far-reaching consequences.

But we already know this. ***Don't We?***

Yet, the biggest worry women have at the first instance of weight gain is about the impact it would have on their appearance.

This misdirected fear of fat goes beyond the boundaries of age, race, ethnicity, education, and social class. It is a psychological barrier most of us have created in our minds. By the time we are able to understand the real consequences, we are already on a perilous one-way street without u-turns.

Obesity is not only a big problem in itself, but it also comes as a package deal. It brings along a number of comorbidities like diabetes, PCOS, heart diseases, depression, stress, and high blood pressure. The list can get pretty big because if you look closely, you'll find obesity as a related cause in most of the 900,000 preventable deaths reported in the US annually.

It isn't that most women don't recognize the issue already; the problem is that most women aren't looking at it in the **Right Context**.

For most women, diabetes, heart problems, high cholesterol, high blood pressure, strokes, are the problems of a distant future. Most women feel that these problems happen to others. These are the problems of the middle-age or even better 'the Old Age.'

They are right to a great extent in the **Wrong Way.**

- It is correct; you won't get diabetes the next day of eating a bag full of sugar.
- It is an absolute fact that high cholesterol buildup doesn't happen in a day. It is a result of years of recklessness.

Most of the diseases we have discussed so far are chronic in nature. They take years, sometimes even decades, to develop. It all starts with a single symptomless problem. It would keep causing the damage. It would keep pushing other systems out of balance. It takes anywhere between

10-20 years for the first chronic illness to fully demonstrate its monstrosity. However, other comorbidities would be quick to follow.

When these chronic illnesses finally hit, people simply fail to understand what just happened to them, but by then, it is literally too late.

Do you know that 4 in 10 adults in the US had more than one chronic disease?

Did you also know that this rate is much **HIGHER in Women**?

A Scientific Fact:

Women are susceptible to gain fat. Their bodies are designed in a way that they tend to gain fat much faster. Even the natural fat percentage in a woman's body is much higher than that of a man's body. This is the cost of having the power to bear a child.

However, this also increases the risks:

The percentage of obese men, including extremely obese men in the US, is 35%. However, in women, this percentage is 40.4.

The rate of extreme obesity in men is 5.5%, whereas, in women, it stands at 9.9%.

In their 40s and 50s, around 38% of men are obese. The percentage for obese women in this age group is 42%.

Would you be surprised to know that in the US, 69% of all the women over the age of 20 are overweight or obese? The percentage of women with an envious hourglass figure is only 8%.

It is understandable that being a woman can be tough sometimes. There is a lot to handle. Yet, missing the fact that 1 in 5 women dying in the US has obesity as the main cause can be a lot to miss.

The sad part is, this is not the end of it.

In the year 2015, there were more than 30.3 million people with type 2 diabetes in the US alone. In fact, in the same year, 1.5 million new cases of Type 2 Diabetes were found. The women easily defeated men, even in this. There were 787,000 women and 743,000 men in newly detected diabetic patients.

Studies have found that diabetic patients have a 53% higher risk of heart diseases. However, that study also reported that diabetic women have a 50% higher risk of heart disease than men.

PCOS (Polycystic Ovarian Syndrome) is a common problem in women in the US. It also has a strange relationship with obesity. Studies suggest that 80% of women with PCOS in the US get overweight or obese. Studies also support the observation that overweight or women have a higher tendency to develop PCOS. This is an area in which women naturally have a monopoly and hence no competitive figures to be drawn.

Obesity is a serious health risk, and it increases the risk of other disease manifolds.

Obesity and diabetes work hand in glove. Obesity creates an even higher risk of heart diseases. The number of triglycerides or free fatty acids in the blood increases due to a high amount of fat production, and that causes a lot of damage to the heart. High blood pressure is another problem that springs up with obesity. The unpleasant bulge created by obesity at the belly and other undesirable areas is an old problem that persists as ever.

- Some women clearly know most of the health risks of Obesity.
- Some women know some of the risks of Obesity.

But how many of you know:

Obesity is just an Effect and not the Cause of the Problems

Obesity simply gets most of the blame because it has a visible presence. It may be behind most of the health complications these days, but obesity in itself occurs due to the malfunction of some very important functions in the body. Till the point, those issues are not addressed, obesity will remain a big problem for you. No matter how hard you run, diet, or repent, the fat would remain adamant.

The first part of this book will help you in understanding some very important things that usually remain missing in the weight loss discussions.

1. Why whatever you eat seem to get added to your fat bulges?
2. Why is it so hard to lose weight?
3. What are the reasons for endless weight relapses?
4. What causes fat gain in the first place?
5. Why does the waist circumference remain the same, although your weight goes down during calorie-restrictive diets?
6. What makes body fat so dangerous for the heart?
7. Why obesity and diabetes create a double whammy?
8. What is the relationship between diabetes and PCOS, and how this book can help you in dealing with PCOS?

And a much more.

Chapter 2: What Makes Us Obese?

The Fundamental Problems

Obesity is a complex problem. There can be several factors that can make a person obese. Some factors are beyond our control, like the contribution of genes. Genetic factors can play a crucial role in making a person fat.

There are factors that lead to temporary obesity like pregnancy. When a woman conceives, the body starts accumulating fat at a much faster pace as it is a great requirement. But, this fat can be made to go away. Most women are unable to do that due to various reasons.

Some women can get fat due to various hormonal issues, but they can also be handled to a great extent, but sadly, they remain ignored. However, the most common reason for obesity blatant abuse of food and lack of physical activity.

We will now try to understand the basic issues that lead to obesity in women.

The Major Reasons

Hormonal Changes

In a woman's body, the hormones play a very crucial role. There is a very delicate balance of hormones in play, and if that balance gets disturbed, it can lead to a number of problems like issues with the menstrual cycle, difficulty in conceiving, infertility, and weight gain. However, before you tie all your obesity woes to hormonal issues, it is important to understand the hormonal problems that lead to obesity and what causes them.

In this chapter, we will be discussing these hormonal issues in brief and explain to you the problems they cause. We will be discussing them in greater detail later in the book and would also explain the impact of intermittent fasting on those hormonal imbalances.

- **Insulin- The Fat Storage Hormone**: Imbalance in this hormone can be the harbinger of problems. This is one of the most dominant hormones that lead to obesity. It is behind most of the catastrophes like obesity, PCOS, and diabetes. However, before you start making a dark image of this hormone in your mind and begin cursing it, remember that it is also one of the most important hormones in the body. This hormone helps the cells in the body in absorbing glucose for survival. It also stores excess glucose as fat. Without this hormone, the body cannot survive. It is a hormone that your body badly needs but at a steady rate. When the body stops producing this hormone in the required amount, you get diabetes. When your body stops responding to the signals of this hormone, you get insulin resistance. Insulin resistance is the single most important reason for obesity. Poor eating habits, unhealthy foods, and a sedentary lifestyle are some of the things that lead to insulin resistance. The good news is that insulin resistance can be reversed. The hard fact, without treating insulin resistance, you can't get out of the trap of obesity. Intermittent fasting is the most reliable way to reverse insulin sensitivity.

- **Leptin- The Satiety Hormone**: This hormone is a hormone produced by the fat cells in the body. When someone has eaten the required amount, this hormone instructs the brain to stop eating by making the body feel satisfied. However, inflammation in the fat cells can affect this mechanism, and the person may never feel satisfied with food. It is a problem with which many obese people will identify. It is not their hunger for food but the inability to feel satiety that leads to this problem. It is a big reason behind keeping you tied to the vicious cycle of obesity.

- **Growth Hormone- The Fat Burner Hormone:** The body produces this hormone in large quantities at younger ages as it is required to aid growth. However, one of the qualities of this hormone also includes faster fat burning. As we age, the production of this hormone goes down. In certain conditions, the production of this hormone can completely stop, and that can make fat burning very difficult. Excessive presence of insulin can also inhibit the production of Growth Hormone and make fat-burning difficult, also leading to obesity. Intermittent fasting can help you in increasing the production of growth hormone in the body.
- **Cortisol- The Stress Hormone:** This is a hormone that the body produces when it is experiencing any kind of stress. The stress can be physiological, psychological, or emotional, but if the stress persists for long, the impact of this hormone on the body would be detrimental

nonetheless. This book will help you in understanding the ways in which this stress can be brought down by following intermittent fasting.

Poor Eating Habits: This is an easy one. We all know that poor eating habits can lead to obesity. Some women simply can't seem to control the amount of food they eat and the kind of reliance they have on food. They don't treat food as a means of survival but also latch on to it for mental and emotional support. This kind of eating can be dangerous, and it will certainly lead to obesity. There is a general misconception that eating your fill in a regulated manner can also lead to obesity, and that's why most women end up on severe calorie-restrictive diets which are punishing at the least. As I already mentioned, it is a misconception. Eating as per the body's requirement doesn't cause obesity; it is a need. However, overeating is a problem that needs to be addressed. We will be discussing it in detail further in this book.

Poor eating habits include two major things:

Overeating: Overdoing anything is harmful, and eating can be no exception. The extra calories that you consume finally end up being stored as fat. However, the story of obesity is far deeper here.

Overeating and the tendency to eat again and again have darker consequences. Overeating can lead to various hormonal imbalances in the body. It causes insulin resistance and leptin resistance, and hence accumulation of fat increases.

Eating Frequently: It is not the amount of food you eat that causes the biggest damage but the frequency with which you eat it. Frequent consumption of meals creates a big problem for the whole energy absorption mechanism and causes insulin resistance in the body.

Junk Food: Again, no brainers for guessing that junk food would lead to obesity. You can never consume junk food cautiously, period. It is full of sugar, salt, and trans fat. It leads to cravings. It simply takes control of your discretionary powers. You simply can't have enough of it. It will certainly make you fat. There is no safe limit of eating junk food.

Over Consumption of Sugar: This is one part we will be discussing in detail in this book. Sugar is one of the most harmful things that will certainly lead to obesity. We already get the required amount of sugar from natural food sources. Refined sugar consumed in any form only damages our system and leads to obesity. Eating sugar in food products or drinking sweetened beverages only fills your body with empty calories that cause severe damage and lead to food cravings. You would have cravings, and you'd want to consume them again and again. Studies have also found that sugar can be highly addictive, and our brain gets hooked on to it.

Lack of Physical Activity: Physical activity helps in burning calories faster, and hence it is a great way to burn fat. A sedentary lifestyle slows down the fat-burning process and it also leads to various health issues.

Genes: This is one area in which you have little control. We inherit the genes from our ancestors, and they can make us prone to weight gain. However, most people use genes as a shield for their weight gain. It is correct that certain genes can make you susceptible to weight gain, but that doesn't mean you can't do anything to counter that. Correct diet, lifestyle, and proper management can help you in ducking this problem.

Diseases: There are several diseases that can lead to weight gain. For instance, PCOS makes weight gain much faster. Diabetic patients also start gaining weight quickly.

There are several physical and mental disorders that increase the tendency of a person to gain weight.

Medications: There are several medications that can lead to weight gain. It is always better to be aware of the side-effects of the medicines you are consuming and work in the right direction to avoid the problems caused by them.

Stopping Breastfeeding Early On: This is also an issue that can lead to weight gain. It has been noted that the women who breastfeed for longer are able to lose weight faster. The women who stop breastfeeding early on tend to retain the fat and find it hard to melt that fat later on.

Misinformation: Wrong information is also a big cause of obesity. Obesity is a widespread problem, and it is also behind several other health issues. Therefore, it is natural for people to seek its solution. However, most of the time, the information that comes through the web is not accurate, or the reader has no means to correctly understand or apply that information and it can also lead to obesity. Aggressive marketing by the food-producing companies also leads to misinformation. Various food product advertisements shout at the top their voice that fat is bad, but none of them says that they use Sugar to compensate for the loss of fat in their products and it is even worse than fat. At one time in the past, even the government advised people to consume more carbs for good health.

Obesity Is Not the Cause of the Problem- It is a Consequence

There is a general misconception that we get unhealthy because we have got obese. In fact, it is the other way around. You get obese because there were underlying health issues that were getting ignored for long, and fat accumulation is just a consequence of those problems. If you want to fight obesity, you will have to understand that obesity is not a cause but an effect.

Let us look at some of the major health issues:

Diabetes: Diabetes is a debilitating health problem. People simply identify it as a problem in which the body is unable to produce insulin in an adequate amount and hence faces problems in blood sugar level regulation. However, Type 2 Diabetes, the most common type of diabetes, starts as insulin resistance and creates a big problem in the fat storage mechanism. It is not your obesity causing diabetes, but the factors that lead to diabetes also lead to obesity. Reversing insulin resistance can save you from both diabetes and obesity at the same time.

Cardiovascular Issues: People wrongly believe obesity to be the main cause of all their cardiovascular problems. It is correct that obesity would lead to heart issues, but it never begins like that. High blood sugar, high blood pressure, and excessive amounts of a free fatty acid called triglyceride in your blood cause the problem. Behind all these three issues, the biggest factor is insulin resistance.

High Blood Pressure: High blood pressure can harm you in a big way. It is bad for the heart, kidneys, and the brain. Insulin resistance is a big reason behind high blood pressure in the body.

High Cholesterol: High cholesterol and high bad cholesterol like LDL (Low-density lipoprotein) and TGs (Triglycerides) to be very specific are the biggest reasons behind most of the heart damage. Insulin resistance contributes in a big way towards increased production of both of these bad cholesterols.

Chronic Inflammations: Inflammations that run for unreasonably long periods can be very bad for the body. The main cause behind inflammations is undue stress on the body, unhealthy lifestyle, overactive immune system, and poor quality food. It also leads to obesity. Inflammation in fat cells is one of the main reasons behind poor appetite control among obese people. It can be treated with a healthy diet and intermittent fasting.

PCOS: The cysts in the ovaries can make the life of a woman very difficult. They lead to weight gain, poor blood sugar management, pain, irregular periods, infertility, and other such issues. It has been scientifically proven that insulin resistance is one of the biggest reasons behind PCOS.

The body works as a unit. If one function is getting affected, other functions would inevitably get affected. These processes are so closely linked with each other that it is difficult for people to identify the right culprit. Most of the reasons that lead to obesity are silent in nature. They keep damaging your body and seldom have a direct impact. When the fat starts appearing, it is visible, and hence people take it to be the primary cause of the problem.

It is very important that you identify the main culprit correctly, and then only the problem can be addressed accurately.

Have you ever wondered why people have to stay on punishing diets for months, and yet they don't lose any significant fat? It happens because they are not addressing the right issue. In most of the cases, it is insulin resistance that causes the problem. If you try to get rid of obesity without trying to reverse insulin resistance, the end result would be a failure.

Chapter 3: Why Do We Fail?

Insulin Resistance- The Devil in the Hiding

Have you ever wondered the reason for failing to lose weight even after trying so hard?

Does it bother you that no matter what, the belly fat stays there adamantly?

Has weight relapse become a curse even for you?

Even when you are starving yourself through those punishing calorie-restrictive diets, the belly fat never seems to budge.

Do you know the reason, why?

We are trying to solve the obesity problem in the same way as Christopher Columbus tried to find the far east, by going in the wrong direction.

It is a clueless search of answers.

Calorie restrictive diets are the preferred medium to lose weight. Women get on these diets and deprive themselves of regular food for months. In the beginning, they lose some weight. They feel elated. They feel that the diets are working. This gives them the required push.

However, after some time, the progress gets stalled. The weight loss stops. They have to get off a diet after a certain period, and that's when the real damage starts. They start to gain weight. Sadly, some women gain even more than what they had actually started with.

The reason is...

When you get on a diet and start reducing your calorie intake, the body gets into a crisis management mode. Everyone has a specified energy need. Consuming less than that makes the body think that something has gone wrong. It starts reducing the energy needs to manage within the current supply. It starts shutting down all the processes that consume excessive energy but are not important for survival.

One such process is temperature management.

Our body retains a lot of water in order to maintain a comfortable temperature. However, it also uses a lot of energy. When you get on a calorie-restrictive diet, the body gets rid of this excess water so that it can save energy. This is called a water dump. This is the reason people start losing weight rapidly when they get on a calorie-restrictive diet.

However, it is also a big reason for such reason to start feeling unreasonably cold or hot. That water was providing them the required comfort.

When you are on a calorie-restrictive diet, you also start feeling weak and lethargic. This happens because the body is trying to conserve as much energy as possible.

Even though the weight goes down a little, people seldom see a reduction in their waist circumference. The reason is their inability to burn down any fat. Calorie-restriction lowers the body's rate of energy consumption. However, it doesn't lead to fat burning. Fat burning is a completely different process. The body would burn fat only as a last resort. This can only happen when the body completely stops receiving energy from external sources. Without cutting off the energy supply completely, it is not possible to hit the fat stores. If you lower the rate of energy supply, the body would only lower its energy requirements to match the supply. It wouldn't hit its treasured fat stores.

This is exactly what happens when you practice severe calorie-restriction. Your body lowers its energy demands to match the supply. The lethargy and loss of energy you feel is simply a result of that energy conservation.

However, in this whole process, no fat burning takes place. No actual weight loss is there. Whatever weight loss is experienced, it is only the water weight that will come back as soon as you resume a normal diet. This is the reason weight relapse is so fast.

The body is still at the same stage. The only thing that you have lost is your energy and will.

Now, the Important Question Is:

Why is burning fat so difficult?

Fat burning is so difficult because you are not providing the right environment for fat burning. This is where insulin comes into play.

Before we get back to fat burning, you must understand the role of insulin in this whole process. It will also explain the way insulin resistance develops and the way it wreaks havoc on your health.

Insulin

Insulin is one of the most important hormones in the body. It is an anabolic hormone. It has two key roles to play in the body.

1. It helps the cells in absorbing glucose in the bloodstream.

2. It normalizes the blood sugar levels by storing excess sugar in the body as glycogen, fat, and free fatty acids.

   It Is the **Main Fat Storage Hormone**. Till there is a high insulin presence in your blood, the body would remain in a fat-storage mode. It will not start burning fat for producing energy.

The Energy Storage Mechanism of Insulin

- The body processes the food and breaks down the nutrients
- It quickly converts the carbs into glucose
- It then releases the glucose into your bloodstream
- The glucose is the fuel your cells can consume directly without any further processing
- The pancreas in the body senses the sudden rise in the blood glucose levels
- One of the jobs of the pancreas is to produce a hormone called insulin to ensure that your blood glucose levels remain stable
- The cells can use glucose in its present form, but they can't absorb it directly from the blood

- The insulin acts as a key to the lock that could help them absorb glucose
- The cells can absorb glucose only in limited quantities as they don't have the capacity to store much
- If your blood sugar level is still high, the insulin would then begin storing this sugar as glycogen and fat

This is the whole energy storage mechanism

Ideally, the calories consumed should be equal to your caloric needs. This is usually not the case.

We live in an era of food abundance. Our eating habits have become such that we consume food all the time. There are snacks after snacks several times a day. We like to eat while we watch TV. We like to eat while we sit to have a chat with someone. We like to consume calories when we are happy. We like to eat when we are feeling sad.

All this leads to excessive consumption of calories, and this happens repeatedly several times a day.

This is the root of the problem.

Repeated intake of food causes frequent insulin spikes. The insulin level in your blood continues to remain high, and this makes the cells slow to the insulin signals. This problem is called insulin resistance. This is what leads to obesity.

Let us understand this in detail. This is the **Most Important Part of the Problem**.

Development of Insulin Resistance:

Insulin resistance isn't a condition you develop overnight. It is a problem caused by the constant abuse of food.

- When you consume food, it is converted to glucose
- This glucose is then absorbed by the cells
- Insulin acts as the key stimulator in the process
- Without insulin, the cells can't absorb glucose
- Every time the glucose levels in your bloodstream go up the pancreas starts pumping insulin
- The pancreas signals the cells to absorb glucose so that the blood sugar levels can be brought down
- But, if you consume meals frequently, the cells will already have plenty of glucose
- They will not be in a position to absorb any more glucose

- The insulin will keep sending signals to them as forcing them to open up
- It becomes a nagging routine. The cells stop responding to the insulin signals
- They start resisting insulin
- This is the **Beginning of Insulin Resistance**

At this level, several things are taking place at the same time, and everything would add up to the problem.

1. The cells stop responding to the insulin signals. Hence the blood sugar levels would start remaining unreasonably high for unreasonably long periods.
2. The cells wouldn't be able to absorb energy readily, and hence they would keep feeling energy starved. Your energy levels would go down.
3. The pancreas would keep sensing high blood sugar levels, and hence pumping of more and more insulin would take place. The cells which were already fed up with high insulin will have more insulin to deal with. This condition is called Insulinemia. This will make them resist insulin even more.
4. Almost all the calories consumed by you will be converted to fat.

Insulin resistance is a condition created by the habit of having frequent meals.

You must understand:

- Anything, however small, if it releases even a few calories will invoke an insulin response from the pancreas
- This means that even if you have a sweetened chewing gums twice a day, that will make two instances of insulin response
- Drinking any kind of sweetened beverage, few morsels of food, pop-corn, diet soda, chips or for that matter anything that releases even a few calories would invoke insulin response
- After any insulin response, it takes around 8-12 hours for the insulin levels to go down
- Therefore, if you have the first calorie response at 8 in the morning and last around 10 at night, your body will never be able to experience a period when the insulin levels go down
- This will lead to **INSULIN RESISTANCE**

For a second, just leave out all the calories you have been consuming in the day. Although they also have a deep impact, for now, let us forget them and focus on this problem.

Simply consuming too many meals a day will also lead to obesity, irrespective of the number of calories you consume. Even if you are consuming a fewer number of calories than the requirement, the problem would be the same for you. Remember, the cells wouldn't respond to the insulin signals. They would need the energy, but they wouldn't be able to absorb it, and hence most of the calories you consume would get converted to fat.

This is the Main Cause of Obesity. It is also the main reason for calorie-restrictive diets to fail.

Insulin, besides being a messenger to the cells, is also the main fat-storing hormone. It is anabolic in nature. In means, it has a tendency to build up fat. This implies that till your body has a high insulin presence, no matter how hard you try, you will not be able to lose weight.

This is another reason people are unable to lose weight even after trying so hard.

The real sign of any progress is a reduction in waist circumference.

You must never take mere weight loss as a sign of progress. If you want to see if you are actually making any progress, you must use the scale as well as the tape at the same time. There may be times when you may be gaining weight on the scale but losing inches on the tape. This is the time when you will be making real progress.

This happens when you are actually burning fat but gaining muscles in place of fat. The fat is voluminous but doesn't weigh much. Whereas muscles are compact but weigh more. That's the reason you may weigh more, but the waist circumference would go down, and this is a sign of great progress. This is the kind of result you should expect while following intermittent fasting.

To Sum Up:

- Insulin resistance is the main reason behind obesity and other related disorders
- Eating at frequent intervals is the main cause of insulin resistance in the body
- Insulin resistance will make losing body fat impossible

- It will also lead to a number of other health disorders

Chapter 4: What is Intermittent Fasting?

It Isn't a Diet

Intermittent Fasting is a very simple concept of purposeful eating in a controlled manner. It is a timed approach to eating food. In this method, you follow periods of fasting and feasting within the same day. You can consume 2-3 meals within the feasting/eating window in a day. During the fasting period of the day, you wouldn't be consuming anything that contains calories. This also includes sweetened beverages or anything else that has calories.

In this approach, you will have to follow two very simple rules.

1. Within a day, your fasting periods would be longer than your feasting periods.
2. You would solely rely on nutritious meals and remove the habit of frequent snacking

Following Intermittent Fasting

Easy Food Rules

Following intermittent fasting is very simple. It isn't a diet, and hence it doesn't set very hard and fast rules for food items.

It is understood that a major reason for weight relapse in the calorie-restrictive diets is the temptation for food that builds up due to severe restrictions. Once the restrictions are lifted, the dieters simply want to have all those food items that they were deprived of. This leads to binge eating, and hence all the effort they had put up in the past month gets washed down in the drain. A complete restriction will lead to longing, and that is not very healthy either for the body or for the mind. Intermittent fasting doesn't impose any such food restrictions.

It is easier to think that you wouldn't be making such mistakes and would refrain from reckless eating after getting off a diet. However, when you have been experiencing such food deprivation since long, most other things become irrelevant. It all starts with taking a small bite and then temptation takes over.

Intermittent fasting doesn't impose any such restrictions on the practitioners. You can eat virtually anything during your eating windows. It is desirable to eat 'not so very healthy items' only in very small quantities, but there is no need to completely abandon them and keep longing.

For instance, if your coworkers are celebrating something and you have been invited, you don't need to keep desiring and drooling over the cake lying at the center. You can have a small piece of it. It is not a very healthy thing to eat, and hence it would be wise to eat it only in small quantities. Eating such things even in smaller quantities puts a stop to the unending yearning of the mind.

In a woman's body, it is not the gut but the mind that longs for such food items. Deprivation of food can cause anxiety, frustration, anger, and depression. It is a big reason calorie-restrictive diets lead to mood swings in women. Food provides solace and security. Putting long-term restrictions on food can start making the mind feel insecure.

It is important that you remove the junk food, high sugar foods, sweetened beverages, chips, cookies, crackers, bagels, and other such items from your routine life.

However, the process needs to be gradual, and it shouldn't create a feeling of longing and desperation. Intermittent fasting allows you the time to bring this change gradually. You can begin by limiting the portion size of such things first and then move on to their complete elimination from your diet.

The Feasting and Fasting Windows

Every day you will have to fast for a certain period of time. For women, fasting for 14 hours is ideal. It helps them lose weight fast, and it also doesn't come in the way of their hormonal balance.

Most people think that fasting is a very difficult task, and they may not be able to follow a fasting routine. The beauty of intermittent fasting is that it is never too heavy on the practitioner. Given that they bring this change gradually. If you think that you would be able to practice the whole routine perfectly from day one, then you are wrong. However, if you make the transition slowly, intermittent fasting is the easiest way to burn fat.

The greatest part of the fasting routine passes away while you are still in your sleep, and hence there are no hunger pangs or cravings for the most part of it. The last leg of the fasting routine falls in your wake time, but that can also be managed with a healthy routine. If you follow it up with a correct diet, there will be no hunger pangs at all.

Women get a feasting window of 10 hours. This window gives them the liberty to pass the whole active and working day without the restriction of fasting.

You can have the first meal of the day at 9 in the morning and the last meal of the day at 7 in the evening.

Simply sticking to this schedule of not eating in the remaining 14 hours of the day can have amazing health benefits. Fat burning and weight loss would become easier than you could have imagined.

What Makes it Effective

The first thing that makes intermittent fasting so effective is its **ability to Reverse Insulin Resistance** and bring insulin sensitivity.

The main cause of insulin resistance in the body is the overexposure of insulin to the cells. The higher the number of meals you consume, the lower will be the duration between meals. It means that your cells wouldn't get a chance to rest. The insulin would continuously keep knocking at their doors for glucose absorption.

The modern lifestyle has become such that we tend to take dinner late at night. Some people even like to work late at night and have coffee, sweetened beverages, or alcoholic beverages. This means that their body never really gets more than 6-8 hours between the last and the first meal. This keeps their insulin level always very high. Remember that it takes at least 8-12 hours from your last calorie intake for the insulin levels to deplete.

Intermittent fasting helps in bringing regulation into their eating patterns. Even a gap of 14 hours will help the insulin levels to go down completely for a few hours. This gives a great boost to insulin sensitivity. The cells become more responsive to insulin signals.

A 14-hour break from any kind of calorie intake means that your body would experience extended periods of an energy crunch. The cells will not have glucose at their disposal for absorption, and hence your body will have to metabolize the energy reserved in the form of fat for filling up the energy gap. This whole process leads to fat-burning.

The absence of insulin from the body also gives way to the production of certain fat-burning hormones that can't be produced in the presence of insulin as the main job of insulin is fat storage. When insulin is low, the body can produce these hormones like the Growth hormone and adrenaline that can aid fat burning.

Sustainability

One of the biggest problems with most weight loss methods is that they aren't sustainable in the long-run. It means that no matter what kind of calorie-restriction you are following, you can't continue it forever. You will have to discontinue it after a certain point.

The Key Reasons are:

The Results Get Plateaued: Calorie-restriction diet results get plateaued after a time. The reason, the body continuously tries to make adjustments to that level of calorie intake. It finds a balance and stops feeling the need to dump any more water weight or shut down any other process. As far as it is possible, the body would like to keep the fat stores undisturbed. The fat reserves are the fuel for the future when there is a complete energy blockade.

Long-Term Food Deprivation Can Lead to Temptations: Anyone who has been on a diet understand the pain of food deprivation. Even if you never had the lust for certain foods, diets make you long for those items as you are completely barred from eating them. This deprivation acts against our very nature and leads to problems. Temptation leads to binge eating. Food simply becomes irresistible. This is the reason people tend to gain more weight than they had lost.

Hormonal Imbalance: For a woman, food is much more than a means of sustenance. A woman's body is tied with a very delicate hormonal balance that can get affected by long-term calorie restriction. This can cause several health problems.

Side Effects: Anger, frustration, irritation, giddiness, lightheadedness, irregular menstrual cycle, and painful periods are just some of the problems that can arise if a woman stays on a calorie-restrictive diet for very long.

It is not a sustainable way to lose weight. You can follow a diet for a few weeks or months at the most but not in continuity. Various surveys have demonstrated that within a year of ending a diet, more than 80% of people who get on diets end up gaining more weight than they had started with.

Intermittent Fasting- A Way of Life

Intermittent Fasting, on the other hand, isn't a diet. It is a way of life.

Sustainability: You slowly shape your routine in a way that fasting for 14 hours becomes a part of your life. This makes the routine very sustainable. There is no deadline attached to it. After a certain point, you stop feeling as if you are doing something out of the ordinary. It becomes an integral part of your life. Your life becomes more balanced, effortless, healthy, and stress-free.

No Food Cravings: The usual way of eating may look more relaxed and comfortable, but it isn't. The body is constantly looking for something more fulfilling and satisfying. That happens because the cells are not getting energy due to insulin resistance. Anything that you eat doesn't fully get to the cells. This leads to frequent hunger. The snacks we have in our diet are full of refined carbs and sugar. They lead to insulin spikes, but the energy is shortlived. Soon you'll start feeling the cravings again. When you rely on 2-3 balanced meals consumed in intermittent fasting, cravings go away. The correct composition of macronutrient helps you in feeling satiated for longer. It is low on carbs and high on fat and protein. This means that the food will get processed slowly, and not only your gut would remain engaged but the food will also keep releasing energy at a steady pace. Your cells would keep getting energy at a steady rate and hence there wouldn't be energy cravings. This brings greater satiety. We will be discussing this in detail in later chapters.

Fat Burning: Intermittent fasting creates the right conditions for fat burning in the body. When there is a high presence of insulin in the blood, no fat burning can take place as the body is in fat storage mode. Remember that insulin is an anabolic hormone. However, when your insulin levels go down in the fasting windows, it creates the perfect environment for the production of fat-burning hormones. This is a reason you will actually witness the belly fat burning and your waist size going down.

Intermittent Fasting Isn't A Magic Pill

There is no doubt that intermittent fasting has emerged as an easy way to lose weight and burn fat. However, that doesn't mean that it comes without consequences. It is not a magic pill that can solve all the health issues faced by you. Following intermittent fasting is a comprehensive lifestyle change. It would require substantial lifestyle changes that may not be suitable for everyone.

If you think that you can simply begin fasting without understanding the complete process and the important things, then there can be dangerous consequences.

A very important thing to understand is that intermittent fasting isn't a treatment. It is a way of life. So, if you are suffering from any kind of health disorder, you must consult your physician before beginning intermittent fasting.

It is a comprehensive lifestyle change. It would bring definitive changes in your eating habits and diet; this means that if you are suffering from any chronic condition, it can have an effect on it. You must discuss this with your physician in advance.

In case you are on long-term medication, you must consult your physician before beginning intermittent fasting as it can affect your health. Long fasting hours can affect your medication.

In case you are suffering from blood sugar management issues or diabetes, you must consult your physician. Intermittent fasting can lead to longer and sustained dips in blood sugar levels that can be dangerous for people suffering from diabetes. You must understand that although high blood sugar levels are dangerous, even low blood sugar levels can be equally devastating and fatal. You must consult your physician as a dose adjustment of your medicines may be required. The physician may also like to monitor your blood sugar levels more frequently.

In a nutshell, Intermittent Fasting is the way to keep a healthy body healthier for much longer without the use of medication. In case you are suffering from any long-term ailment, you will also require the guidance and supervision of your physician to assist in the process.

There are some important things that you must remember:

Intermittent Fasting is a way of life and not a treatment

It would require a long-term commitment

You would need to be faithful to the routine

The results can be slow, as it may take you some time to adjust to the schedule.

The best results will only be seen when intermittent fasting is coupled with a nutritious and balanced diet and exercise.

Intermittent fasting against the medical advice of your physician can be dangerous. If you are not suffering from any chronic health disorder, intermittent fasting can help you in staying healthy for long without the use of medicines. However, if you are suffering from any health problem, consult your doctor first. Explain your routine so that the doctor can help you in making that routine possible.

Chapter 5: Practicing Intermittent Fasting as a Woman

The Hormonal Conundrum and Shorter Fasting

One of the aspects of being a woman is having to deal with a delicate hormonal balance. In a woman's body, there are several important hormones at play. Besides other things like growth and development, these hormones also regulate fertility, metabolism, and the ability to bear a child. These hormones make all the difference there is, to have a woman's body. They differentiate a woman from a man. They dictate physique, emotions, mood, libido, and even the ability to have kids. However, it all comes at a cost. The complex yet delicate hormonal balance makes the body of a woman more sensitive to external stimuli.

Relationship with Fat

A woman's body is more inclined to accumulate fat. This is a scientific fact, and there are strong reasons behind it. A woman's body likes to store more fat than an average man because it always likes to keep itself prepared to fight with adverse conditions of energy shortage.

Since the time a girl reaches puberty to the time she achieves menopause, the body of a woman is always prepared to bear a child. However, childbearing isn't something that the body can take lightly. It hoards fat in order to support the process. Fat is a very important source of energy, and hence it is treated as a prized possession by the body. It will fight tooth and nail against every effort to get rid of the excess fat. The fat is treated in the body as a counter-measure against energy shortages.

In case, there is an acute shortage of energy while a woman is pregnant, the body doesn't want to leave everything to chance. It hoards a substantial amount of fat in advance so that in case of emergencies, problems can be averted as far as possible.

The body doesn't know when you can get pregnant as hence it simply likes to keep the extra fat all the time.

This is the reason the healthy fat ratio in men is between 8-19%, whereas the same ratio in women is between 21-33%.

It has been found that the Oestrogen hormone in women is the key to excess fat storage. It makes them susceptible to easier fat storage and makes losing fat difficult.

A Strong Attachment to Food

Women also have a very strong attachment to food. This attachment is not with the quantity of food but its availability. When you bring sustained calorie restriction in your life, you are effectively sending a message to your body that there is a situation of emergency. The body doesn't take this lightly; it starts making changes in your menstrual cycle as well as your ability to bear a child. It can also have a deep impact on your mood and emotions. You may become more irritable, temperamental, and also start having frequent mood swings.

Experiments on rats have shown that the mice that were subjected to calorie-restriction had shrunk or smaller reproductive organs as compared to the ones who weren't subjected to such changes. Affected mice also behaved in an erratic manner and became more aggressive.

Similar things have been observed even in women. Therefore, it is advised that women shouldn't undertake severe calorie-restriction as it can alter their hormonal balance.

Even with fasting, women need to tread very carefully. If you are suffering from hormonal issues, you must consult your doctor before beginning any kind of fasting. Men can do longer fasts with little or no impact on their health. In fact, it has been observed in various studies that intermittent fasting helps men in reversing their insulin resistance pretty quickly.

However, that's not the case with women. If you have just started experimenting with intermittent fasting, you must **Never Start With Longer Fasts**.

It is very important for women to start with shorter fasts and help their bodies get accustomed to the change. It is only when their body gets used to a certain fasting period that they should choose to move further.

The attempt should be made to find an intermittent fasting routine that can help them in losing weight faster without affecting their health and hormonal balance. Ignoring this simple yet important thing can have far-reaching consequences, and that's why it is important that men and women fast differently.

Intermittent Fasting Isn't Calorie-Restriction

On the face of it, you may feel that both have uncanny similarities. They deprive the body of food and energy in some way or another. However, this is the point where you are wrong.

Intermittent Fasting doesn't affect your calorie intake in any way. You will be free to have a reasonable amount of food during your eating windows. This means that within the 2-3 meals that you will have, you can consume an adequate number of calories. The only different thing would be that you'd still lose weight. While following intermittent fasting, there is no need to eat less or consume fewer calories. Intermittent fasting is not about what to eat but when to eat. It tries to correct the way energy is being used in the body.

The biggest cause of obesity is the inability of the cells to utilize the glucose present in the bloodstream. When this glucose isn't absorbed by the cells due to insulin resistance, the insulin has no other option than to store it as fat, and this leads to fat accumulation and obesity.

Intermittent fasting helps in the reversal of insulin resistance. This means that the cells in your body will be able to use the available glucose, and you will feel more energetic and healthy. There will be less glucose floating in the body to be stored as fat, and hence fat accumulation wouldn't remain a problem.

The longer fasting windows help in creating shorter energy crisis situations that force the body to metabolize the stored fat. In this way, even the stored fat starts to go down.

Calorie-restrictive diets, on the other hand, create systematic energy deprivation that makes the body become defensive of its fat stores. In place of using the fat stores, the body starts reducing its calorie needs to ensure that it can last longer with the stored energy. This is the most logical thing to do from an evolutionary perspective, but as far as burning fat is concerned, it will make burning even a gram of fat difficult.

The highest blame for obesity is easily put on high-calorie intake. 'Overeating is the cause of obesity.' This is a statement that's difficult to defend. However, does that make an statement like this a universal truth?

There are several qualifiers that are missing in this statement.

Overeating, while leading a sedentary life will cause obesity. Overeating is a necessity if you are doing hard labor, you are a sportsman, you do high-intensity workouts.

Overeating and doing that several times a day at frequent intervals will cause obesity. This will lead to frequent insulin spikes, and the whole insulin balance will get off, causing obesity.

Overeating too many simple carbs will lead to obesity. When you eat too many items made up of refined carbs like white bread, chips, cookies, cakes, bagels, etc. your blood sugar levels keep getting spiked after short intervals. This is a sure-shot recipe for insulin resistance and will lead to obesity.

Your body is well-equipped to deal with usual transgressions. When these transgressions become a norm and start taking place with impunity, obesity is a consequence.

You must remember that obesity is not the cause of the problem; it is a consequence of bad eating habits and poor food choices. It can be corrected by following a healthy lifestyle and proper eating routine.

Intermittent fasting presents a simple and straightforward solution to most health issues that people face these days. It is a practice that's easy to follow and helps your body to gain its natural pace.

It not only helps you in burning fat and fighting obesity, but it also helps you in getting rid of a number of health issues.

The next chapter will help you in understanding the problems you may face due to obesity and the ways in which intermittent fasting can help you.

Chapter 6: Health Benefits of Intermittent Fasting

By now, it would have become clear to you that intermittent is just not a weight-loss method. It is a method to bring a holistic change in overall health. It simply helps you in fixing the inherent health issues that lead to obesity. Once the problems are resolved, the body doesn't find it difficult to deal with the obesity problem.

We have several processes going inside the body that work on their own. For instance, the liver has its specific functions. The blood circulation also works on its own. The same goes for most of the processes running in the body. However, the body works as a unit, and if one process starts working against the body, it has a deep impact on your overall health.

Let us assume that a person is suffering from high blood sugar levels. Now, this means that the blood would get thick and hence moving the blood to various parts would get difficult. This will have an impact on your blood pressure levels.

High blood sugar also leads to high cholesterol accumulation.

It would also affect the kidneys. High blood sugar levels start blocking the kidneys, and their efficiency in purifying the blood goes down.

High blood sugar also means that your blood sugar levels would remain high; this high concentration of insulin can adversely affect the ovaries and cause PCOS. When the insulin levels in the blood are very high, they lead to an androgen shift. This androgen shift then causes PCOS.

High blood sugar would also mean that the insulin present in the blood will be under immense pressure to stabilize the blood sugar levels. However, when the cells are not responding and absorbing glucose, the insulin starts converting the blood sugar into free fatty acids or triglycerides to be stored in the body as fat. This causes high cholesterol and high triglyceride problem. This process would also kickstart the process that would lead to chronic inflammations.

This was just to demonstrate the ways in which a single problem can lead to a number of health issues. It is very important that you don't just run after visible issues like obesity and ignore the underlying problems that are causing it.

Intermittent fasting is a way to bring holistic changes to your health. It will help in improving the overall health biomarkers so that you can attain optimum health. Weight loss and fat burning would be the byproducts of this positive change.

Some of the Immediate Health Benefits of Intermittent Fasting are:

Improved Insulin Sensitivity

We have already discussed the importance of insulin. It is the key anabolic hormone that's responsible for fat storage and obesity. However, it is also a crucial hormone for your survival. The problem begins when your body stops responding to the crucial insulin signals.

The pancreas gets overworked as it has to pump more and more insulin for the same job. The cells get more annoyed as they have to deal with more and more insulin than required. The blood glucose levels remain unreasonably high. This is a mess your body is not very pleased to bear.

Intermittent fasting can help you with this problem. In fact, intermittent fasting is the best way out of insulin resistance. Several studies have proven that limiting calorie intake for certain periods in a day can help in improving insulin sensitivity.

Studies conducted on a number of people practicing day-time fast during the festival of Ramadan have proven that it is an effective way to improve insulin sensitivity. The tests conducted on the participants demonstrated lower blood sugar levels. Their cholesterol levels also improved, and it did help in bringing down the body fat.

When you observe fasting for 14 hours and above, your insulin levels go down considerably as there is no instance of an insulin spike. This means that the cells get a chance to be in an environment that's not overcrowded with insulin. This is the single biggest reason responsible for reversing insulin resistance and bringing insulin sensitivity.

It is the best environment for the production of fat-burning hormones.

Faster Fat Burning

A protruding belly is not a desirable state for any woman except when she is expecting a baby. However, it is a state in which most women find themselves nonetheless. Accumulation of fat at the belly, hips, and thighs is very common. This fat is the hardest to burn. We now understand the reasons this fat is so adamant.

Insulin resistance is a key player in the accumulation of fat in the body. It is the key fat-storage hormone. If there is a high amount of insulin in your blood, the adipose tissues will keep storing fat. It doesn't matter the amount of hard work you put forward; your weight loss would be slow. The reason is simple; the body is in fat-storage mode. However, you may wonder about the things that may happen when the insulin levels go down.

Does the fat burning start automatically?

Unfortunately, nothing happens on its own in this body. But, low insulin levels trigger the production of various hormones that can speed up the whole fat burning process. There is a hormone called the Human Growth Hormone or the Growth Hormone, as it is popularly called. This hormone is responsible for many things in the body, fat metabolization or burning fat is one among them.

This hormone has some of the most amazing qualities. It will not only burn fat in the body but would also prevent the loss of muscle mass. This is a bonus. All those people who might have undertaken any kind of high-intensity exercise in the past know that working hard helps in burning fat, but it also leads to the breakdown of a lot of muscles in the process. With the Growth hormone present in your body, you can be sure that, for the most part, you'll only be burning fat.

Production of Growth Hormone requires some special conditions:

1. The insulin levels in your blood should be very low
2. Its production is high during sleep
3. A bit of hunger accelerates the production of this hormone

With the help of intermittent fasting, you will be able to meet all the requirements mentioned above. Due to a 14 hour fast, the insulin levels in your blood would be really low. As the fasting windows are usually scheduled to take place at night, you will be fast asleep when this takes place, and hence it would help in the production of the growth hormone. By the time the production of growth hormone starts, your stomach is usually empty and hence there is a presence of the hunger hormone called ghrelin.

This means by the time you wake up, your body will have an adequate amount of growth hormone. Studies have shown that intermittent fasting can help in increasing the production of growth hormone several times over. Even following intermittent fasting for a few days can bring an increase of 300% in your growth hormone production. Studies have demonstrated that with the help of intermittent fasting, the growth hormone production in women can go as high as 1300%, and in men, it can go up to 2000%.

At the same time, the production of adrenaline also goes up in the body, and both these hormones help you in exercising hard and burn the calories faster. This is a reason it is always advised to exercise in the morning as this is the time the level of growth hormone and adrenaline is high in the blood. It will fetch much better results. You will be able to burn many more calories by exercising in this state rather than in any other condition.

Better Blood Sugar Regulation

High blood sugar is a cause of several problems. At the beginning of the chapter, we have understood through the example the kind of damage high blood sugar can cause. High blood sugar is caused by only one reason, and that is an inefficient use of sugar. If your body is not producing a sufficient amount of insulin, there will be high blood sugar. This condition is called Type 1 Diabetes. This condition is genetic, and you can do nothing about it. However, it is rare, and only 5% of people suffering from diabetes in the US are suffering from this condition. The second type is called Type 2 Diabetes; in this condition, your body loses the ability to respond to insulin properly. It is caused by insulin resistance and it is the most common type of diabetes.

The pancreas has the responsibility to produce insulin. It is a very efficient gland. However, it can get overworked due to our poor eating habits.

When you eat anything, your body converts that food into glucose. This glucose is released into the bloodstream. Every time glucose is released into the bloodstream, the pancreas starts pumping insulin to manage the high blood sugar levels. This creates an insulin spike in your bloodstream.

If you keep having frequent meals at short intervals, the blood sugar level in your bloodstream will keep increasing as the body is already struggling with the management of the previous glucose.

The pancreas keeps sensing high blood pressure, and it just continuously pumps insulin in the blood. This makes the insulin levels go very high. This situation isn't going to help you in any way.

Once the insulin is released into the bloodstream, it takes anywhere between 8-12 hours for the insulin levels to go down.

The higher the number of meals you consume, the greater the amount of insulin in your blood. This is what makes insulin resistance even worse.

The habit of having frequent meals and snacks is very dangerous for blood sugar levels and the pancreas.

Intermittent fasting helps your pancreas by creating longer fasting windows in which the pancreas doesn't have to produce insulin. In this window, the insulin levels in the body also go down, and hence the cells also get a chance to develop a bit of insulin sensitivity.

Both these processes combined help in keeping the blood sugar levels down.

Normal blood sugar levels are not only good for your weight management, but they also help in maintaining normal blood pressure and a healthy heart.

Lower Risk of Heart Problems

Heart problems are a big risk in obesity. The number of women succumbing to heart problems is much higher than men. If there is diabetes, the risk of heart problems goes up considerably. A study noted that obese women with diabetes had a 50% higher risk of heart attacks compared to men.

The biggest cause of heart problems is a higher percentage of bad cholesterol and a lower percentage of good cholesterol.

High-Density Lipoprotein is considered as good cholesterol, and it can clear the plaque from the arteries and bring them back to the liver for further metabolization. Low-density lipoprotein is considered as bad cholesterol as it sticks to the artery walls and narrows its diameter. It also reduces the flexibility of the arteries making the required expansion and contraction difficult. There are times when this plaque deposited inside the walls breaks apart and causes blockage of heart. It can also make the arteries weak and cause leakage in them.

There is another kind of bad cholesterol called triglyceride. This is a free fatty acid that your body can use as energy, but it keeps traveling freely in the blood and gets deposited in the heart. In the case of insulin resistance, insulin starts converting glucose directly into triglycerides to normalize the blood sugar levels, and this escalates the problem. When there is visceral fat in the body, it also leads to the production of a lot of free fatty acids.

Intermittent fasting helps you in putting a break to the whole process. It helps in lowering the production of triglycerides by better management of blood sugar. It also helps in bringing down chronic inflammations in the body that also prevents heart problems.

Lower blood sugar levels also help in normalizing the blood pressure levels, and that is again good for the heart.

Improved Satiety

This is a very important point that gets missed most of the time. Most obese women have very poor control over their appetite. In fact, most obese people have very poor control over their appetite. This simply means that they find it very hard not to eat something. Most of the time, when they eat, or they are offered food, they aren't really feeling very hungry, but they find themselves simply unable to resist the temptation to eat. The food is never really able to satisfy them completely. This is a reason they overeat most of the time. If you think that it happens due to poor self-control or lack of determination, you are wrong. This happens because of inflammation in the fat cells. We call this problem Leptin Resistance.

Leptin is a hormone released by the fat cells in the body. The job of this hormone is to signal the hypothalamus in the brain to instruct you to stop eating. The hypothalamus makes you feel satisfied with the food and brings satiety.

When you are hungry, the gut releases a hormone called ghrelin. This is the hunger hormone. This hormone increases your tendency to eat food. Ghrelin and Leptin are the opposites. When you feel hungry, the ghrelin levels are very high, and the leptin levels are very low. However, as you eat, the ghrelin levels start going down. This makes you feel less and less hungry. At the same time, the ghrelin levels start increasing. As you eat, the energy starts going inside the fat cells, and they start increasing the release of leptin. This hormone signals the brain to stop eating and bring a feeling of satiety.

However, when insulin resistance persists for long, it leads to various inflammations in the body. It also inflames the fat cells in the body. When the fat cells are inflamed, they lose control over the release of leptin. The fat cells start releasing leptin at a moderate rate all the time. This means that you are eating or not; the fat cells would keep releasing leptin. This leads to overexposure of the brain to this hormone. It becomes resistant to the leptin signals.

This means that either you are eating or not, the rate of release of leptin is the same. The brain stops registering these signals. It means that when you are actually eating anything, the bain doesn't get to know that you are full. It never releases the signals of satiety, and that's why obese people are not able to resist food and stop eating.

Intermittent fasting helps even in this situation. It helps you in eradicating snacks from your routine, and hence the habit of frequent eating goes away. It also brings longer periods of fasting. The long absence of food in the system helps the fat cells in managing the leptin release. Intermittent fasting also helps in fighting chronic inflammations in the body, and that is also very helpful.

Chronic Inflammation

Chronic inflammation is another problem that concerns all of us. Chronic inflammations can take anyone their cover. However, there are certain conditions that increase the risk of chronic inflammations several times.

The risk factors are:

- Obesity

- Sedentary Lifestyle
- Poor Diet
- Stress

These risk factors are enough to elucidate the fact that all of us have some risk of chronic inflammation. The obese people are at a greater risk as more than one condition applies to them.

Chronic inflammations are very hard to deal with, as they do not have symptoms. You wouldn't feel a thing until a particular system has got considerably compromised.

Chronic inflammations can cause all sorts of problems, including brain damage. One of the biggest risk factors of chronic inflammations is obesity. The excess fat in the body leads to a constant release of free radicals that lead to oxidative stress and chronic inflammations.

Intermittent fasting can help you in fighting chronic inflammations by bringing down the fat in the body. Intermittent fasting is one of the best ways to burn body fat. Intermittent fasting, coupled with a keto diet, leads to the rapid burning of body fat. The free radicals in the body start getting utilized as the fuel for providing energy, and hence the risk of oxidative stress goes down. Adding anti-inflammatory food along with intermittent fasting and keto can be the best way out of chronic inflammations.

PCOS

PCOS or Polycystic Ovarian Syndrome is a common problem that most women encounter sometime or the other. This condition can lead to difficult or irregular menstrual cycles, fertility issues, excessive male hormones, unwanted hair and hair loss, and small follicles on the ovaries.

One of the most common causes of PCOS is insulin resistance. Obesity is also a big cause, and PCOS also leads to obesity. If insulin levels during PCOS remain very high, there is a great possibility of developing diabetes.

Science believes that there can be many reasons behind the occurrence of PCOS, and there isn't a great clarity about everything. However, medical science is very certain that insulin resistance has a very big role to play in it. Due to excess insulin in the blood, the hypothalamus and the pituitary glands in the brain get affected and begin releasing androgen hormones. This causes the androgen shift. Due to the impact of excessive insulin, reproductive glands begin producing masculine hormones like testosterone in larger quantities. This causes unwanted hair growth, PCOS, and other such problems.

Excessive release of androgens is a very big problem in itself. It can also lead to infertility and ovarian dysfunction. This can happen with or without having PCOS.

Insulin resistance is a very big problem. It can bring a host of problems. In fact, even in PCOS, the problem of obesity increases the complications. However, it has been seen that PCOS is also responsible to a great extent for causing obesity.

The Conventional Route and Its Failures

As you can see, Insulin Resistance is the root of the whole problem. It is behind every single problem that you face, and obesity is simply one among them. However, it is also a problem that somehow remains undiagnosed for years, although the signs are always there. The doctors ask do blood sugar tests and even the HbA1c to check the average blood sugar of the past 3 months. But, it is seldom that patients are asked to get HOMA-IR to know the actual state of insulin resistance.

Even when Insulin resistance is diagnosed, the doctors put the patients on Metformin or similar medications. These are insulin sensitizers, but they don't solve the problem of insulin resistance; they simply try to hide the symptoms.

Insulin resistance is a problem originating from long-term lifestyle disorders. It isn't something that develops overnight. Years of overuse and abuse of food, unhealthy lifestyle, lack of physical activity, and chronic stress lead to the problem.

If you really want to get out of the clutches of this problem for good, then you will have to bring substantial changes in your lifestyle and eating habits, as well as your diet.

Intermittent Fasting is the right step in this direction. It is a simple and easy way to get out of the vicious cycle of obesity and insulin resistance and the pack of problems these problems unleash upon us.

Intermittent fasting has proven to be a really successful way to reverse insulin resistance and bring insulin sensitivity. It also helps in getting rid of obesity and brings a positive change in other health biomarkers.

However, the problem is that most people get overenthusiastic at this point and forget that intermittent fasting is no magic trick. In fact, it is going to be a very tight rope walk as a woman. The delicate hormonal balance in the body of a woman never allows the liberty to take things easy. You have to remember that you must start slow and follow all the instructions carefully.

Chapter 7: The 16/8 Intermittent Fasting Protocol

The Process and Preparation

Intermittent Fasting- Sustained Benefits

The 16/8 intermittent fasting protocol is one of the most popular approaches in intermittent fasting. It has several distinct benefits.

First, it is easy to follow. One of the best things about this intermittent fasting protocols is that it can be easily followed and turned into a lifestyle. This is also one of the most important things. Most of the problems that arise like obesity, insulin resistance, high blood pressure, and heart problems develop because of a poor lifestyle. There can be no quick remedy or a one-time solution for these issues. Even if you are able to miraculously get out of these issues with the help of some medication or help, these problems can again develop if you don't bring a change into your lifestyle. For anything to work, it is important that it can be followed for longer periods, and intermittent fasting perfectly fits into this description.

Second, it doesn't require a tectonic shift or big compromises. One of the biggest reasons for the failures of various diets and other weight loss measures is that they require a big change. Because you are so desperate for a solution, you bring those changes immediately. However, it is always very difficult to maintain any significant change that's against your nature for a very long period. Food is a necessity and also a habit. Cutting into it can be asking for a lot. This is a reason diets start looking torturous after a period of time. In this aspect, intermittent fasting is a cakewalk. It doesn't ask you to make a substantial change in your diet. It simply asks you to abstain from eating for a certain period of time. It is not a very difficult thing to do as, for the most part of that period, you are fast asleep. You get the time to make small but definitive changes in your eating and fasting habits.

Third, it starts showing real results quickly. Nothing can motivate a person more than results. Intermittent fasting is no doubt a bit slow in showing results, but still, within a fortnight, you would start experiencing signs of improvement. The changes experienced are not only in terms of weight and waist circumference but also in your overall health, which you can experience within.

You will start feeling more energetic. The lethargy goes away.

Most insulin-resistant people usually feel drowsy after having a meal in the afternoon. It is a sign that your body is struggling in processing energy. This goes away quickly as your insulin sensitivity improves with intermittent fasting.

You also witness improvement in your mood and temperament. This happens because your body is no longer dependent upon the kick it used to receive from the insulin spikes. These are just some of the things that you will experience.

The overall experience of intermittent fasting is rejuvenating.

Following intermittent fasting can quickly bring you back on the track. It helps you by restoring insulin sensitivity and burning fat deposits. These are the two big troublemakers in the body.

Be Warned

One of the biggest mistakes women make while beginning intermittent fasting is that they do it in haste.

They want to have all the benefits from the word 'Go.' Sadly, life doesn't work that way. These issues didn't arise all of a sudden, and hence there is no way to make them go just like that. Even if you do the hardest routines, you will be standing at the same place even father back.

Unfortunately, many practitioners don't pay heed to this advice, and they have to pay for this mistake later on in the form of hormonal imbalance.

Intermittent fasting is a major lifestyle change. It is a long-term commitment, and you must ensure that your transition to this lifestyle is as smooth as possible, and only then you can expect complete success.

Tread Softly

The best way to begin intermittent fasting is to take baby steps into the process.

It is understandable that you may not feel the need to move slowly. Afterall you are free to eat almost everything during your fasting windows and then remain in a fasted state for the duration a bit longer than your sleeping hours. How difficult can that be?

This happens when people don't fully understand the gravity of the process and also when they are overzealous. However, this can be a big mistake.

Given below is the reality check of every part of the routine.

1. You Can Only Eat 2-3 Meals in a Whole Day

Yes, this is to bring some clarity about the eating window. You will certainly have a 10 hours window in the 16/8 intermittent fasting routine, which for women is 14/10. In the 10-hour long eating window, you can only have 3 meals at the most. Besides these three meals, even a can of diet soda is also not allowed. You will have to put a complete stop to all kinds of snacks, beverage breaks, tit-bits, and munchies. Anything besides 3 meals will be out of your reach. Now, imagine yourself passing the whole day without the help of those things. I hope this will help you in getting a grasp of reality.

2. The 14-Hour Long Fasting Window Can Start Looking Very Long

This is something people don't realize in the beginning. Passing 14 hours without food for an uninitiated person can become very hard. It is something to which you have to get used to. It doesn't come on its own. You may feel a bit constrained. You may want to cheat one day, and then it would become a habit, and the whole routine would fail for you. You will have to learn to fast for 14-hours and train your body to do that.

3. Physical Exercise Is A Must

Intermittent fasting, all the fat metabolizing hormones, and the improved insulin sensitivity only pave the way for fat loss. The actual and significant fat loss would only take place when you really do some intense physical exercise. You can't leave everything on fasting alone.

You Must Prepare

The keyword to success with this routine is to prepare. It is very important to prepare your body and mind for the initiative you are going to take. If you just had to fast for a day or a week, maybe this kind of preparation wouldn't have been necessary. But, intermittent fasting is a long-term commitment, and you wouldn't want your body to scream all the time to get out of the routine. The best way to avoid this problem is to slowly prepare yourself physically and mentally for the schedule.

The Preparation

First Step- Eliminate Snacks

This is one of the most important and even the hardest of the steps. The snacks we eat during the day are not needed by the body. If we eliminate them from our diet, nothing substantial will change. But, they have become such an integral part of our lives that doing so becomes very difficult.

If you look closely, we have at least 6-7 snacks in any given that. Here, I want you to include all the instances when you consume sweetened beverages like coffee, soda, or any kind of alcohol too. Each of these things would add calories to your system and hence would cause an insulin spike. Therefore, these things would have to be eliminated. Then eliminate every other kind of snack that you have. If you like chewing gum, that would have to be stopped. If you like taking coffee breaks, that will go. If you are fond of protein bars in the day, they would also need to go. The kind of snacks you like can be different, but they would have to go.

This is a troubling part, and it may take some time for you to get used to it. However, there is no way out of it.

If you want to get success in fat loss, you will have to do away with snacks. A word of caution, do not move ahead with intermittent fasting until you have gained considerable success in eliminating the snacks from your routine. Don't just feel this in your mind, but practically follow it for a few days and try to acclimatize yourself to the change.

Start with 12-12 Routine

Once you have eliminated snacks from your routine, start with a 12-12 routine. This simply means that you will have 12 hours of fasting window and 12 hours of eating window. You can space your meals at an interval of 4 hours each for the sake of convenience. There is no hard and fast rule for this. It's just that keeping them spaced equally helps in managing hunger better in the beginning.

In the beginning, you can even keep your fasting windows shorter than 12 hours. If it works for you, go for 14 hours of eating window and 10 hours of fasting. This is just for the beginning phase when you are just learning to maintain complete abstinence from food for a certain period of time within a day.

Your end goal should be to complete the fasting window without obsessing over food. You can give yourself as much time at this stage as you want. But, only move ahead when you are able to maintain 12 hours of fasting window without any difficulty.

This would become easier with a balanced and nutritious diet as that would help you feel satisfied for longer. We would be discussing that in detail in the coming chapters.

The 16/8 Intermittent Fasting Protocol

For women, this routine is 14/10. It has been observed that women are able to lose weight better even with 14 hours of fasting, and that also doesn't mess with their hormonal cycles. This is a reason this intermittent fasting protocol is 14/10 for women. However, it is still known as 16/8 because both are the same in all other aspects, and 16/8 is quite a popular one and resonates in the minds of the practitioners.

The intermittent fasting protocol is also known as the LeanGains protocol, and there are specific reasons for that. People practicing this intermittent fasting protocol lose their body fat easily but don't lose their muscle mass. This means that this intermittent fasting protocol helps in gaining a lean and muscular body mass. The loss of muscle mass would be less, and the fat burning would be more.

There are several ways to follow this intermittent fasting protocol, and it would depend on what kind of a person you are. For instance, if you are a morning person and like to wake up early, it would be better for you to begin the fast early in the evening. It has several benefits. If you begin your fast early, you wouldn't have to stay hungry for very long in the morning. If you wake up and 6 in the morning and have to wait for breakfast till 10, it can get difficult as there would be 4 hours at the end of the fast. This can be the time when the hunger pangs would be the most severe. The best way out would be to begin your fast around 6 in the evening.

Beginning your fast at 6 means that you will have to finish your dinner at that time. Eating at six will give you several advantages. First, there would be at least 4-5 hours before you go to sleep. This will give your body long enough to digest the food completely before you hit the bed. This will make your digestion system work even better. Going to bed with a belly full of food is a very bad habit, but sadly most of us have been there.

Eating about 4-5 hours before going to bed means that you wouldn't really start feeling very hungry by this time, but the stomach would have started to get empty. This means that insulin levels would soon start plummeting, and the production of the growth hormone can begin early. We have already discussed the importance of this hormone in fat burning.

You can wake up around 6 and then spend the next 2 hours doing exercise and the regular morning things. You can have your breakfast around 8 and begin the 10 hours of the eating window.

If you take pride in yourself for being a night owl, you must postpone your dinner further in the evening to around 8-9. This will help you in staying awake for later without having the urge to eat anything in the middle of the night. The worst thing about having to stay up till late at night is the urge to eat. When you are awake, the digestion system seems to work much faster. That's the reason if you are going to have to stay up late you must consume dinner late. But, it should be at least 3-4 hours prior to your hitting the bed. This helps your digestive system to process the food better.

You need to follow this routine every day. Some people seem to be drawn towards cheat days. They want to have at least one cheat day every week. You' be disappointed to know that taking cheat days gives you body and mind an excuse to break the routine. This becomes a habit, and soon it leads to falling apart of the whole routine.

It may happen that someday you break your fast half an hour or one hour faster and, on other days, keep the fast for a bit longer. But, you will have to stick to the routine on its basic structure.

Exercise Daily

You must exercise every day. It doesn't matter the kind of exercise you do, but you must do it every day of the week. If you feel that your weight is stopping you from doing any kind of rigorous exercise, simply go for a walk. Bringing the body into motion is very important for the fat to start metabolizing. When you do any kind of physical activity, it creates an energy demand that will help your body in burning the fat stores. Staying on the couch all the time can prove to be counterproductive.

Chapter 8: Losing Weight with 16/8 Intermittent Fasting

You Can Do It

A big apprehension in the minds of women is that would they really be able to lose weight and how the process works. This chapter would help you in understanding the way to make intermittent fasting work for you.

Being suspicious of the success of weight loss measures is nothing unusual. Unwanted fat and weight can be a very sensitive matter for a woman. It not only hurts the public appearance of a woman, which in itself is a very big thing but also affects confidence. To get rid of this fat, women try a variety of mediums. The rapid expansion of the weight loss industry to the extent that today it has a market valuation of $72 billion tells the tale.

From exercise and supplements to pills and surgeries, women try everything, but the fat simply stays.

Exercise

Exercise is a great way to lose weight and stay fit, but you simply can't rely on exercise for weight loss. There are some serious issues with this approach. The first and foremost thing is the problem with sustainability. Some women pick up rigorous exercise routines in the beginning, but they're never able to keep up to it in the long run. Life comes in their way. It is one thing to aspire to sweat in the gym to hours daily and entirely something else to practically find the time to do that. A woman's life is also riddled with several responsibilities and the pressures of balancing work and personal life. All this simply never allows that to happen. Even if you are able to do that, insulin resistance will certainly stand in the way of fat-burning. Without creating the right environment inside the body, it is impossible to metabolize fat.

Supplements

Another common way is through supplements. They simply never work for weight loss. Supplements are great for fulfilling deficiencies. If you are on the path of weight loss, the supplements will give you the required push and acceleration. However, if your body is resisting the change in weight, the supplements would simply won't work.

Pills

There are hundreds of TV commercials and other mediums shouting about wonder pills that will burn your fat like magic. If you have ever fallen for them in your life, then you'd already know the truth, and if you still haven't given to the temptation, then consider this a warning. They simply don't work and can even be very harmful. There is no regulation on these pills and they can become a real health nuisance.

Surgery

Surgery is the last resort available to morbidly obese people as it can help you in bringing down your weight. However, you must understand that bariatric surgeries are very expensive and will only be performed by the doctor if your weight has exceeded a certain threshold. Besides that, even the gains of bariatric surgeries can be shortlived if you don't change the ways of your life. Even surgeries involving gastric bypass and sealing off a significant portion of your stomach are only effective for a short term. The body starts adapting to the change, and the weight starts to go up within a couple of years.

Even these surgeries have their own side-effects and may lead to severe nutrient deficiencies and a poor quality of life.

If you look closely, you'll find that these measures fail because you are not providing the right environment to the body for burning fat. Simply pumping iron for hours is not going to fetch results if your body is in continuous fat-storage mode. Even surgeries won't help you if your lifestyle remains the same as before. The need is to adopt a lifestyle that's conducive to weight loss.

Intermittent Fasting does that for you. It creates the perfect environment for weight loss and fat burning.

How Intermittent Fasting Helps

The first thing that intermittent fasting does is that it puts a stop to your habit of frequent eating. Every calorie intake leads to insulin spike inside the body and would lead to insulin resistance. If you already have insulin resistance, the glucose produced from frequent meals would start getting converted to fat directly. The insulin in the body would be struggling to stabilize the blood sugar levels, and hence it would lead to a direct fat conversion.

With the help of intermittent fasting, you are able to get rid of this dangerous phenomenon.

A minimum of 14 hours of fasting window inside the body will again help in bringing your insulin sensitivity back.

Once your insulin sensitivity returns, your body will be able to process glucose better. A major portion of glucose produced from your meals would start getting consumed by the cells. The remaining would be used by other metabolic processes, and hence in this way, your weight gain would stop. Mind you, intermittent fasting is one of the best ways to maintain an ideal weight, and this is how it takes place. Most people keep struggling all their lives to maintain the lost weight. It is as difficult a process as losing weight.

Burning the accumulated fat is a bit more complicated process than this.

Fat-Burning

If you want to burn fat, you will have to understand the process the body uses for burning fat.

Our body runs on two kinds of fuel:

1. The glucose fuel that you get from carbs and protein

2. The fat fuel that you get from dietary fat and the fat stored in the body

Traditionally, fat was the original medium of fuel for the humankind as we had no knowledge of carbs. Humankind heavily depended on hunting and gathering. The animal meat provided the required amount of fat and protein to our body. The fruits and vegetables gathered provided the small amounts of carbs and fiber that the body needed. Till this time, obesity, diabetes, high blood pressure, and high cholesterol were not the problems of humankind.

We consumed fat in large quantities, and hence our bodies ran on the fat fuel. The fat is a cleaner fuel as it leads to very little toxic waste inside the body. It is very healthy.

Once we started agriculture and farming, our diet changed from predominantly being a fat-rich diet to a carb-rich diet. The carbs are broken down as glucose. It can be absorbed by the cells directly as fuel, and it is easy to break down. Therefore, it became the preferred medium of energy. However, carbs leave a lot of toxic waste inside the body.

Your body can only use one type of food at a time. It means that if your body is running on glucose fuel, it will keep running on glucose fuel till all the glucose gets exhausted. This is the cause of the problem. If our diets remain predominantly carb-rich, our body will face problems in burning the fat as it would require switching the fuel source, and that's something that requires time.

Intermittent fasting gives you the gap in which your body can be free from any kind of glucose, and hence it can burn the fat fuel in the body. It is a long-term fat-burning strategy.

When you start following your intermittent fasting routine, you will be creating gaps in which all the glucose in the body would be over. The insulin levels in the blood would also be minimal. This is the time when your body would have no other option than to burn fat for energy as it requires energy at a constant rate all the time. The fat can be broken down in the liver into ketones that can also power your body.

The longer the fasting period is, the faster would be the fat burning. However, this is the place where women have a big disadvantage as longer fasts can create hormonal imbalance in their body. The 14-hour fast is the middle way that can help you in burning fat without causing hormonal imbalance or any other problem.

The progress may be slow, but intermittent fasting is a steady way to burn fat at a consistent rate. Once your body gets adapted to the change, there will be minimum side-effects, and you will be able to burn fat while feeling healthy. If you make suitable changes to your diet and adopt a healthy exercise routine, the fat-burning pace can be increased and you can experience faster fat-burning.

Chapter 9: The Basic Diet Rules in 16/8 Intermittent Fasting

Understanding the Food Basics- All Calories are Not the Same

Food plays a very important role in health. In fact, 80% of your health is directly dependent on the kind of food you eat, and only 20% impact is created by exercise and other such things. It is our food and eating habits that have led to this health fiasco.

Not very far ago, just a century or so from now, the death rate was very high, but it was due to infections, communicable diseases, wars, hunger, and famines. However, deaths due to metabolic disorders and obesity were rare, if none.

In this age, with the help of science and technology, we have almost conquered communicable diseases. Widespread infections claiming lives in millions are unimaginable for the current generation as thankfully, it has no memory of it. However, obesity, diabetes, high blood pressure, and other metabolic disorders have become commonplace. They are claiming more lives than anything else. These issues have become more common and prevalent than hunger and poverty.

As per the WHO report, more than 1.9 billion people in this world are currently struggling with weight issues.

This is not a very small number. In fact, it covers almost one-fourth of the world population.

The overweight and obesity numbers in the US are even starker. CDC report says that more than 70% or two out of three adults in the US are overweight or obese. Almost 40% of these are obese, also including morbidly obese.

Apart from our poor eating habits, another thing that's responsible for this catastrophe is unhealthy food and poor food choices.

Our food is highly dominated by refined carbs and sugar. The percentage of healthy fats is low, and we are consuming poor-quality protein. All this leads to obesity and poor health.

A major part of our food is the macronutrients. These are the ingredients from which we derive energy.

There are 3 types of macronutrients:

Carbohydrates or Carbs: We get carbs from grains, fruits, vegetables, and all kinds of agricultural produce. Carbs are a major portion of our diet. There are some fruits and vegetables that also have fat and protein content too, but they also have a good amount of carbs in them, and hence you can generalize agricultural produce as carb-rich. All carbs are not bad.

The carbs can be further classified into three categories:

1. **Refined carbs:** These are the bad carbs. We get them from bread, bagels, cracker, chips, high starch foods, sugar-rich items, cookies, candies, and other such products that have sugar and processed grains. These carbs are very easy to process, and hence they get digested very fast, releasing all the glucose at once. They cause the highest amount of insulin spike and consumption of these carbs must be limited if you can't stop it completely.
2. **Complex Carbs:** These are the good carbs. We get them from whole grains, whole foods, non-starchy vegetables. These carbs take a very long time to get processed in the gut and release glucose at a very slow and steady pace.

They don't cause insulin spikes, and hence they are good for your body. The whole grains also contain some important trace minerals that are essential for your growth and development. A bit portion of your carb diet must come from complex carb consumption.

3. **Fiber:** Fiber is the indigestible material that you get from fruits, vegetables, and grains. It is very important for the health of the gut as it helps in cleaning it and restoring the balance in the gut. Consumption of fiber-rich food is also important as it takes a very long time to get digested, and the release of energy is very slow. Food items like whole grains have indigestible fiber that comes out exactly the same form unaltered. It scrub cleans your intestines, and it plays a very important role in your intestinal health. From fruits and vegetables, you get a gel-like soluble fiber that helps in restoring the gut balance. Both these fibers are very important. You must eat fruits as a whole as the pulp is made up of this fiber. Eating non-starchy green leafy vegetables and cruciferous vegetables also give you a lot of fiber along with antioxidants,

phytonutrients, flavonoids, vitamins, and minerals. They also help you in reaching food satiety faster and feeling full for longer after having a meal.

Protein: Protein is a macronutrient that you get from lean meats, legumes, cereals, and dairy products. Protein is important for building muscles. Each day as you go by the normal activities of the day, several muscles break, and new ones take their place. When you do high-intensity exercise or weight training, the rate of muscle destruction and new muscle formation increases manifolds. This is one macronutrient for which your body solely depends on your diet. The body doesn't produce protein. It should be an ideal part of your daily diet. However, you must consume only a certain amount of protein that the body can use for building muscles. Excess protein will be broken down to produce glucose. Including the required amount of protein in the diet will help you in reaching satiety faster. It takes much longer than the carbs to get broken down and releases energy very slowly. This will also prevent insulin spikes and will provide energy at a steady rate. By including a good amount of protein in your diet, you can also ensure that you don't eat, and it will make you feel satisfied much faster.

Fat: Fat is the third and most important part of the diet. It releases more energy per gram and takes much longer to get broken down, and hence eating fat can make you feel satisfied between meals, and you wouldn't crave snacks. Fat also doesn't invoke an insulin response from the body as metabolization and absorption of fat don't need insulin. The alfa cells in the pancreas produce glucagon that can convert fat into energy. Hence, fat-rich foods also lower the instances of an insulin spike. Making fat a major part of the diet can help you in lowering insulin resistance and get sustained energy. It also means that your body will not have to make frequent switches between burning glucose and fat. This will also facilitate faster fat burning.

Carbs, protein, and fat all are sources of energy. We measure energy in calories, and hence it is important to get an idea of the calories they provide.

Carbs provide 4 calories in 1 gram

Protein provides 4 calories in 1 gram

Fat provides 9 calories in 1 gram

Although carbs and protein provide the same number of calories per gram, they are not the same. The carbs get processed very fast, and hence the energy produced by the carbs is short-lived as it gets used up fast. Protein, on the other hand, gets processed very slow, and hence the energy is released at a constant rate. Even the calories provided by the carbs are not the same. The refined carbs lead to an instant insulin spike as they get broken down into glucose rapidly. The complex carbs take much longer and hence produce energy at a very slow pace. Therefore, the complex carbs do not cause an insulin spike of a similar nature. The fat doesn't cause an insulin spike at all as the process of fat breakdown is completely different.

Another category of carbs that we usually consume a lot is called empty calories. We get empty calories from things that cause an insulin spike but don't give anything to the gut to process. Sweetened beverages, fruit juices, energy drinks are some of the examples of empty calories. These are the things that cause the highest amount of damage as far as fat accumulation is considered.

When you ingest empty calories, they get converted into glucose instantly but don't provide anything to the gut to work upon. This creates two distinct problems. First, the gut starts releasing digestive juices in anticipation of food, and when nothing really comes down, these juices get wasted. They also cause damage to the gut biome. Second, a large number of calories ingested through these energy drinks raise the glucose levels in the bloodstream instantly. They cause a severe insulin spike, and the body starts struggling with the management of the blood sugar levels. Insulin has to finally convert all the excess glucose into fat.

Therefore, you see that consuming fat will ultimately lead to a breakdown of fat in the body, whereas consuming refined carbs and sugar-rich food will increase fat in the body.

Intermittent Fasting and Diet Rules

The diet rules in intermittent fasting are simple. You simply need to ensure that the food you consume doesn't lead to a severe insulin spike. It should be such that it provides satiety for longer. If you eat food items rich in refined carbs, they will get processed fast, and your body will not have anything real to process. In that case, you will feel hunger pangs and food cravings much faster, and it would become difficult for you to maintain longer fasting hours.

1. Your diet must have a good amount of protein. It will help you in remaining satiated for longer.
2. The quantity of fat should also be high as it also helps in making you feel fuller.
3. You must consume as much fiber-rich food as possible. Non-starchy green leafy vegetables, fruits with pulp, whole-grain foods, and legumes are some of the things that provide a lot of fiber in the food. It also fills you up fast. Total caloric intake is also low in these things. All these things make high-fiber food an ideal part of an intermittent fasting diet.
4. The refined carbs should be consumed the least as they don't last long and lead to cravings.
5. High sugar food items should be eliminated; they cause insulin spikes and raise your blood sugar levels.

6. Empty calories shouldn't be consumed at all. Don't drink juice, eat the whole fruit instead. Don't drink carbonated beverages, even diet soda or zero-calorie drinks are equally harmful. There is no such thing as zero-calorie if it is sweet. Alcohol is also a big cause of insulin spikes along with other health issues it creates. Consumption of alcohol should also be limited if not stopped entirely.

Chapter 10: The 16/8 Intermittent Fasting Protocol isn't Restrictive

You Can Still Pretty Much Eat Anything You Like

Intermittent fasting doesn't impose blanket bans on food items like most calorie-restrictive diets people follow. Intermittent fasting isn't a diet at all. It is simply a lifestyle change that helps your body in becoming more insulin sensitive and increases the conditions for fat burning.

One big problem with imposing a complete ban on a food item is the longing and temptation it creates in mind. Even if you never liked that food item before now simply because you can't eat it, your mind would create cravings for those food items. This phenomenon becomes many times severe when this happens with the food items that you really like. More often than not, these food items are sugar-rich, and hence they are a strict no-no from the health perspective.

However, weight loss is as much a mental phenomenon as it is a physical one. Suppressed longings for food never allow your mind to rest, and you try to compensate for that loss by overeating or other such equally damaging modes if not more damaging.

Intermittent fasting doesn't put any such restriction. You can eat whatever you want. However, there should be two simple rules.

1. You must eat them well within your eating window
2. You must consume them only in very small quantity and not make it a habit

These two simple rules can help you in avoiding temptations, and you will be able to move on the path of fat-burning without having to curse yourself every step of the way.

Intermittent Fasting is More About 'When to Eat' and Less about 'What to Eat'

Intermittent fasting gives more emphasis on 'when to eat.' This is important as your eating pattern influences the insulin resistance in the body as well as the fat-burning mechanism. 'What to eat' is not a very big issue because if your body is burning energy at a steady pace, then a few extra calories would get burned without difficulty. If your body is facing problems in metabolizing glucose in general, then every extra calorie would be a burden on your system.

However, this doesn't mean that you can overload your system with calories. It only means you must consume a healthy and balanced diet to an extent you start feeling satisfied. Remember that it takes around 20 minutes for the hypothalamus to induce satiety after you have had your fill. This means by the time you feel around 80% full, you have eaten the required amount. If you take a short break at that time, you won't feel hungry at all after a while. This happens because, by them, the feeling of satiety has taken over.

Therefore, you must eat cautiously. You should stop eating when you start feeling even a little bit satiated.

Overeating is not going to help your cause, and hence it must be avoided as far as possible. Try to include things in your diet that take up more space but add fewer calories to your system. For instance, you can include unlimited portions of non-starchy green leafy vegetables in your diet without worrying about the calories. The leafy greens are full of fiber and antioxidants. They have negligible calories, and they can make you feel fuller for much longer.

The 3 Meals of the Day

The 14/10 intermittent fasting routine will give you a chance to have three meals a day. Initially, 3 meals a day should be followed, but as you become more habitual to the routine, it generally comes down to 2 meals and 1 small refreshment of sorts. Having a diet rich in protein and fat has its own perks, and feeling less hungry is one of them.

There are some important things that you must try to follow:

Stretch Breakfast or the First Meal of the Day as Far into the Day as Possible

If you are following the intermittent fasting routine properly and do exercise in the morning, you may not start feeling hungry very early. This will allow you to stretch your breakfast a bit far into the day. It helps you in many ways. If you don't have breakfast very early, you won't feel the urge to eat anything very soon as you'll feel fuller due to the breakfast when you are on the active part of the day. You will feel less inclined to give in to the temptations of snacks and beverages.

Your Breakfast Should be Balanced

Your breakfast should be a good mix of fat, protein, and whole carbs as well as it should have a good portion of the greens. If your breakfast is balanced, your likeliness of feeling cravings for food will go down considerably. Try to avoid starchy and sugary food items completely. If you must have them, don't include them in your breakfast.

You can Have Some Beverages

Intermittent fasting doesn't put a blanket ban on beverages. You can have unsweetened black coffee, green tea, and unsweetened fresh lime water. All these things don't add calories to your system and hence don't invoke an insulin response. Unsweetened green tea is a good source of anti-oxidants, and hence it is good for fat burning. It helps in lowering the rate of inflammations. Unsweetened black coffee will help you in fighting sugar withdrawal symptoms, and it will also help you in suppressing hunger pangs. Unsweetened fresh lime water also helps in suppressing hunger pangs and also helps in speeding up the fat cutting process.

Second Meal of the Day Should Be Light

The second meal of the day or lunch should be light and try to include only the salads prepared at home or leafy greens in your salad as they are light and wouldn't make you feel lethargic. Some people like to have their lunch late into the day and keep it medium heavy. This also helps as it would help you in keeping your last meal of the day even lighter. It all depends on the space you want to keep between both the meals.

The Last Meal of the Day

Ideally, you would be having your last meal of the day early. The last meal of the day should be kept such that it causes the least amount of insulin spike. It shouldn't be very heavy as that can make you feel restless, and you'd want the food to get digested by the time you hit the bed. Keeping it simple and straight is always the best.

The number of calories you want to include in each meal is up to you. In fact, you don't even need to count calories. Simply judge the food by the kind of nutrition it provides and try to keep it free of refined carbs and sugar.

Chapter 11: Calculating the Ideal Caloric Ratio

Mapping Caloric Requirements

Although calculating calories is not a very important thing in intermittent fasting as your body is going to self-regulate itself. You would have to cut down on your snacks, and that will also take away a large number of calories as they have a lot of refined carbs and sugar.

If you stick to 2-3 times a day, you wouldn't have anything to worry about.

Cutting your calorie intake is not a big parameter for fat burning in intermittent fasting.

However, it wouldn't hurt if you consume almost the same number of calories or a few less than you need. You must remember that you shouldn't reduce your calorie intake too much, or else it will have a negative impact similar to calorie-restrictive diets.

If you want to know your required calorie intake, you can follow the given formula.

The first thing to know about your energy needs is to understand your body's calorie needs. This is known as the Basal Metabolic Rate. This is the number of calories your body needs in the idle state. This means that even if you don't do any kind of physical activity, your body would need these many calories to run various processes in the body.

Basal Metabolic Rate

The BMR is calculated by the formulae given below:

BMR: 655+(4.35 x Weight in Pounds) + (4.7 x Height in Inches) – (4.7 x Age in Years)

It means if a woman has the following description:

- Weight 132 Pounds
- Height 5 Feet 10 Inches or 70 Inches total
- Age 32 Years

The BMR Would be 655 (4.35 x 132) + (4.7 x 70) – (4.7 x 32) = 1407.80

These are the number of calories a woman with these particulars would need in the idle state.

If you want to know the number of calories you would actually need, you would have to find out your Total Daily Energy Expenditure.

You can find that out by the formulas given below:

Total Daily Energy Expenditure

Sedentary Lifestyle (No Exercise): BMR x 1.2

Light Exercises 1-3 times a week: BMR x 1.375

Moderate Exercise 1-3 times a week: BMR x 1.55

Very Active Exercise 6-7 times a week: BMR 1.725

High-Intensity Exercise 6-7 times a week and a job involving physical labor: BMR x 1.9

Using these calculations, you can make the required changes in your diet.

Chapter 12: The Keto Diet- Is It The Next Big Thing?

An Intro to Keto Diet

The Ketogenic diet or the Keto diet is another term that remains in big news as far as weight loss is concerned. From bodybuilders to athletes, everyone is talking about this diet.

The word Keto is derived from ketosis. It is the process in which the body starts using fat as the fuel source instead of glucose. It starts breaking the fat molecules into smaller units called ketones, which can be used in place of glucose. The process of using ketones as fuel is known as ketosis.

The keto diet didn't originally start as a fat loss diet. It was designed by a doctor to treat epilepsy in kids, but then other benefits of this diet came into light, and it became a big sensation in the fat loss segment.

The keto diet simply works on the concept of making the body shift its fuel-burning mode.

As you know, our diet mainly comprises of carbs and small amounts of protein and even smaller amounts of fat.

Hence, our body is mainly in glucose burning mode. This process also leads to the release of a lot of toxins.

The ketogenic diet comprises mainly of fat, an adequate amount of fat and a very small amount of carbs. This takes out the body from glucose burning mode and puts it in fat-burning mode. This change in the fuel would mean that once the fat from your diet ends, your body would have no difficulty in burning the body fat for fuel as no fuel switching would be required.

Fat-burning releases a lot of energy, and hence ketosis would make you feel more energetic.

When your body is burning glucose, it experiences several energy dips. This happens because when you consume food, the carbs release a lot of energy instantly. Your body gets into action and starts stabilizing blood sugar levels through various mediums. First, the glucose is absorbed by the cells, and it makes you feel very energetic all of a sudden, then insulin starts storing glucose as glycogen and fat. However, all this needs to be done as fast as possible because the blood sugar levels can't remain very high for very long. The glucose absorbed by the cells can only be used for short periods and hence you would need to consume food again shortly. This is the reason people on high carb diets start feeling hunger pangs so fast.

When your body is in ketosis, there are no such energy dips. Your body first burns the fat in your diet as fuel, and when that is over it starts burning the body fat. Because no energy switch is required, you feel no dips in energy.

This simple principle makes the keto diet one of the best ways to lose weight.

A simple change in diet can make your body more capable of burning fat. This is the reason the keto diet has become so popular these days.

Chapter 13: Keto Diet and Intermittent Fasting

Adding to the Shine

Keto diet and intermittent fasting complement each other perfectly. It is simply a match made in heaven.

Intermittent fasting is a principle that helps your body in creating long gaps so that the insulin in the body can be brought down to its lowest levels. It also leads to the complete depletion of glucose in the bloodstream. Once the glucose levels are down to none, it forces the body to feed on its fat stores for energy.

However, if you are taking a normal diet, the switch would have to be made every day. There would be smaller windows of glucose shortage, and the fat-burning would be slow. But, if you start following a keto diet while practicing intermittent fasting, the body would need to make no fuel switch. It would continuously remain in a fat-burning mode, and whenever dietary glucose supply would go down, the body would naturally start burning body fat.

This is a reason it is always the best to use both keto and intermittent fasting together.

Following intermittent fasting on keto is similar to following intermittent fasting on any other diet. You wouldn't need to make any substantial changes in your routine.

As far as the keto diet is concerned. It can be a substantial change from your regular diet as you will have to make your diet predominantly fat-rich.

The keto diet is High-fat and low-carb. The protein content in the diet is as per the requirement of the body. You must divide the daily protein intake into three equal portions and consume them in your every meal. Do not try to consume all the protein in one meal, as that can also lead to glucose production. Always remember that excess protein is also broken down as glucose. Hence, eating excess protein will harm your fat-loss initiatives.

The carb percentage in a keto diet is very low. It is almost negligible, and the sources from which you can draw your carbs are also limited. This is one big compromise you may have to make. You must draw all your carbs from non-starchy leafy greens and complex carbs. Your diet should be rich in low-starch high fiber food.

If you follow a keto diet with intermittent fasting, you can experience rapid weight loss as a keto diet gives a great push to fat burning. It is important to note that when you are on a keto diet, you can also follow calorie restriction as energy derived from the diet doesn't hold much importance. Your body is burning the same type of fuel, and hence after a point in time when you are in the fasted state, it automatically starts burning the body fat.

Therefore, if your daily caloric requirement is 2000 calories, you can easily bring it down to 500 calories and make the body compensate for the deficit of 500 calories from the body fat. In this way, you will be able to burn body fat faster and also take yourself closer to good health.

Chapter 14: Combining the Keto Diet with Intermittent Fasting

Making Both Work Together

Combining the keto diet with intermittent fasting is the most natural thing to do as both the ideas complement each other perfectly and lead to faster fat-burning besides other health benefits.

The most important thing that you'd need to do is make changes in your macronutrient proportions and implement them in your diet plan.

The ideal macronutrient ratio should be:

Fat: 70-75%

Protein: 20-25%

Carbs: 5-10%

Fat

You should include a lot of healthy fats in your diet.

Healthy fats such as nuts and seeds should make the cut.

You can also include fat-rich fruits like avocadoes.

Grass-fed meats and fatty fish are also good things to include in your diet.

You should exclude fast foods and deep-fried foods. Although they have a lot of fat, the fat is generally trans fats that should be avoided. These food items also have a lot of sugar and salt that you'd like to avoid as they can come in the way of ketosis and are very bad for your heart health and sugar levels.

Although the fat percentage is very high in a keto diet, it doesn't mean that you will have to eat a lot of fat. The fat is high in calories and hence eating even small quantities of fat would make up for the percentage.

Proteins

You can include grass-fed lean meat into your diet for completing the protein content.

Legumes also have a lot of protein, and you can include them in your daily diet. You can eat sprouts as they are a cleaner source of rich protein.

Tofu, cottage cheese, and dairy product, and egg whites also provide protein in good quantities.

Fish are also high in protein, and they also provide Omega-3 fatty acids that are good for your heart.

Carbs

You'll have to be careful while including carbs in your diet. You must only choose high-fiber sources of carbs in your diet. Complex carbs obtained from whole grains can make a part of the carb ratio.

Your focus should be to include as much non-starchy leafy greens into your diet as possible. This is the only type of carbs that you can consume without worrying about the number of calories you are ingesting. You should have at least 7-10 cups of non-starchy leafy green in your diet daily.

These vegetables will fill you up and make you feel satiated much faster. The soluble fiber in these vegetables makes a gel-like substance in your gut that cleans the gut and helps in easing insulin resistance too.

You can also make a puree of these vegetables and consume them.

Anti-inflammatory foods should also be a part of your diet as they help in the chronic inflammations and prove to be an aid in your diet.

Combining keto with intermittent fasting is a simple and effective way to start burning fat rapidly.

Intermittent fasting helps in creating the perfect environment for fat burning, and a keto diet helps in making the whole process faster and smoother.

Chapter 15: The Things to Keep in Mind

Precautions to Take

Don't Be In a Hurry

This is a very important point and can't be emphasized enough. You must not make the mistake of starting with the whole 14/10 fasting routine. This is a very common mistake women make and then end up paying with hormonal imbalance and a feeling of failure. It is important that you give your body the proper time to make the transition.

Our bodies get accustomed to a routine, however bad it is. If you try to change it with a sudden jolt, there can be adverse reactions to it. If you are a person who likes to have smaller food breaks at regular intervals, even a 4 hour-long hiatus from food can start looking much. Your mind would keep pushing you to eat something, and your mind would remain occupied with the thoughts of food. This is something we are trying to avoid.

Therefore, begin with getting rid of the habit of snacking. Once you have got accustomed to that, begin extending the gap between your meals.

First, try fasting for 12 hours and have a 12-hour eating window and then only extend it to 14 hours when your body has fully adjusted to the previous routine.

Listen to Your Body

Always listen to your body. Fasting, even for a bit longer, can have a deep impact on your body. Every woman's body is different. Some women can easily fast for 16 hours and longer without having any kind of side-effect, while there are women who may face problems even in the 14-hour fasting schedule. You must listen to the signals your body is sending.

You must closely monitor if fasting for 14 hours is causing any kind of hormonal imbalance. If your menstrual cycle changes or you face any other kind of difficulty, you must react to that change sensitively.

Try to readjust your fasting schedule to find your comfort zone. Remember that some women may be able to lose weight even with a fasting schedule shorter than 14 hours.

The 14-hour fasting window is not a very hard and fast rule. If you feel that strong hunger pangs some days, feel free to eat something even a bit early.

Some hunger is good for health as it helps in the production of various helpful hormones. It also leads to the creation of positive stress that is healthy for the body. However, you shouldn't overstrain the body as that can cause chronic stress, which might become a cause of fat gain, and that would be counterproductive.

Avoid Sugar

This is something you will have to eliminate from your diet. Refined sugar is something our body is unaware of. It comprises of glucose and fructose. Our body can use glucose directly, but it can't metabolize fructose. This is the kind of sugar that can only be broken down in the liver. Our liver is the second largest organ in the body, but it has the responsibility of performing more than 500 functions and it is the main detoxifier. Breaking fructose is an added responsibility that can get the liver overworked. You must try to avoid that in all circumstances.

The food processing industry has instilled great fear of fats in our minds. Most people believe that eating fat would make them fat. This is the reason most popular foods in the market are fat-free foods. We simply want to throw out fat from every healthy food we eat.

Most of the unhealthy food items are laden with unhealthy transfat that should be eliminated, but we allow it as a guilty pleasure.

The food processing industry has substituted fat with sugar, and that is the biggest health disaster. The fat also adds taste to the food, and when the fat is taken out of the food, it also makes the food tasteless. To compensate for the loss of taste, these companies add copious amounts of sugar in the foods. They even use high-fructose corn syrup in foods which is an even more concentrated form of fructose. These things cause even greater damage to our liver and also lead to frequent glucose spikes and insulin resistance.

You must get rid of refined sugar in your diet. If you have a sweet tooth, rely on the natural sources of sugar like fruits. The fruits also have some amount of fructose, but our body is able to metabolize it easily and doesn't face that much stress.

You must never drink fruit juices instead of the whole fruit as that removes the pulp and fills your system with empty calories. Fiber must remain a big part of your diet.

Maintain a Healthy and Active Routine

If you want to burn fat rapidly, then you must maintain an active schedule. Try to exercise and remain active in your day to day life. Try to take stairs in place of lift as much as possible. If you have a desk job, try to take short breaks and walk for a few minutes.

Go for walks in the morning and evening.

Walk as much as possible, and whenever possible, ditch the car if going nearby.

Stress is another factor that leads to weight gain. The stress hormone can act as a sledgehammer on your system and may slow down the functioning of all other hormones. Try to live a stress-free life. Meditation and yoga can also help you in bringing down stress in life.

Adequate Sleep is Important

Sleep is very important. Your body carries out a lot of repair and maintenance work while you are fast asleep. Depriving yourself of sleep can come in the way of these processes. 7-8 hours of sleep is important for the body to remain in a completely relaxed state. The fasting can also add a bit of stress to the body for which sleep is important.

Your body produces hormones like ghrelin, adrenaline, and the growth hormone, which are helpful in burning fat. If you don't sleep adequately, the production of these hormones will get affected.

Exercise Regularly

Exercise is a great way to stay healthy and create an energy demand for the body, which would be fulfilled by burning fat. Doing high-intensity interval training is the best way to expedite the fat-burning process. You can do High-intensity interval training on non-consecutive days and do simple cardio exercises on the rest days. This would create an ideal fat-burning environment.

Exercise should be done in the fasting state as, during this period, the amount of growth hormone and adrenaline is high in your body. Both these hormones provide stamina and also lead to faster fat-burning. You will have the best results in this period.

If you can't do high-intensity exercise due to excess weight or other health reasons, you must do light cardio exercises. Yoga, running, walking, and swimming also some forms of exercise that anyone can do irrespective of the health constraints.

It is important that you maintain an active lifestyle if you want to bid excess weight good-bye from your life.

Chapter 16: When not to Fast

Respecting The Special Circumstances

Intermittent fasting is an amazing way to attain superb health and avoid the dangers of lifestyle disorders common these days. However, fasting is not for everyone. As I have mentioned earlier, too, intermittent fasting shouldn't be treated as a weight loss diet or a cure. It is a healthy lifestyle. It is something that should be adopted by people who are not suffering from any chronic illness. Such individuals can expect a healthier life and lower risk of metabolic disorders with aging.

If a person is suffering from any kind of chronic illness, intermittent fasting shouldn't be done without the advice of a health practitioner. Intermittent fasting is a big commitment. It can come in the way of your medication or other routines. You must talk to your physician before taking up intermittent fasting.

If you are suffering from blood sugar management issues or diabetes, intermittent fasting shouldn't be done without the supervision of your physician. It can lead to severe dips in the blood sugar levels, which can be dangerous.

Women with a history of eating disorders like anorexia, bulimia, and binge eating should avoid intermittent fasting. Even if you have recovered from these issues, fasting can push you back into these disorders.

Women struggling with anxiety and depression shouldn't practice intermittent fasting without consulting their physician.

Girls below the age of 18 shouldn't fast as it can come in the way of their growth and development. The energy requirements in the growing age are very high, and hence they should avoid practicing it.

Women who are trying to conceive shouldn't practice intermittent fasting. Fasting can affect the ovulation cycle, and they may experience difficulties in conceiving.

Pregnant women shouldn't practice any form of fasting at all. It can be very harmful to both the mother as well as the child. Pregnant women have enormous energy requirements, and fasting can come in its way.

Lactating or breastfeeding women also shouldn't fast.

In case you are experiencing serious changes in your menstrual cycle, you must stop fasting and consult your physician immediately.

If you notice the changes mentioned below, you must stop fasting and consult your physician immediately:

- Rapid and abnormal weight loss
- Heavy hair fall
- Constant irritation
- Persistent dizziness
- Cystic Acne
- Decreased glucose tolerance or insulin sensitivity

These issues are not common, and very rarely does someone experiences these symptoms due to fasting; however, it is always better to safe than sorry. You must remain watchful of these symptoms, and if they appear, consult your physician immediately. These symptoms can also be warning signs of some other serious health issues that might have been developing silently.

Chapter 17: The Possible Side-Effects and the Ways to Deal with Them

Knowledge is Power

Headaches, Lightheadedness, Nausea, and Irritation

At the beginning of the fasting routine, you may experience symptoms like headaches, lightheadedness, nausea, and irritation. These are common symptoms and shouldn't create any panic in your mind. These aren't the problems created by fasting or the Keto diet but by sugar withdrawal symptoms.

When your diet is primarily composed of sugar, the body gets used to frequent insulin spikes. However, when you begin fasting or switch to a sugar-free high-fat diet, it can make your body crave sugar and create such symptoms. There is nothing to worry about as these symptoms will subside shortly. A better and easier way to deal with these issues is to have unsweetened black coffee or green tea twice or thrice a day. These stimulants will help with the headaches and would also make you feel fresh.

One important thing to remember is that you must not rely on these stimulants excessively. Don't drink tea or coffee more than 2-3 times a day as you can start getting addicted to them.

Shakiness and Sensitivity to Hot and Cold

This is also a common problem that you might experience while practicing any kind of fasting. It also happens because the body is used to frequent glucose spikes, and that stops all of a sudden. These symptoms should go away in a few days. You might develop high sensitivity to hot and cold as the body would dump some water in the beginning. However, it wouldn't persist for long as your calorie intake wouldn't change substantially.

Excessive Urination and Mineral Deficiencies

This is a problem that will cause trouble in the beginning. The body tries to adjust itself to the changes in the diet and energy consumption, and in the process, it starts dumping water. This will lead to excess urination.

Although the loss of some water may not be a big cause of concern, loss of minerals can lead to mineral deficiencies. Loss of minerals should be taken seriously, and simply drinking plenty of water doesn't solve the problem.

The main minerals that are lost in the process are:

- Sodium
- Potassium
- Calcium
- Magnesium
- Phosphate

Mineral deficiencies can be overcome by consuming plenty of electrolytes. You can get these electrolyte solutions easily, and that should solve the big part of the problem easily.

Hunger Pangs

In the beginning, you can have hunger pangs. Light hunger pangs are not bad. You shouldn't eat as and when you start feeling hungry. The main hunger hormone ghrelin is released by the gut periodically as it has more to do with routine than actual hunger. If you are feeling slight hunger pangs, then drinking a glass of lukewarm water or lukewarm water with few drops of lemon juice will help you significantly. Responding to every hunger pang is not necessary. If hunger pangs are severe and they become a regular affair, then you may have to adjust your diet and make it more nutrient-dense.

Food Cravings

Food cravings are primarily caused by sugar-rich foods. If you are consuming a high-carb diet, the chances of food cravings will be high. These cravings get even worse after you have eaten sweets or other such things that are full of sugar. The best way to avoid food cravings is to stay away from sugar and sweets.

Heartburn, Constipation, and Bloating

Heartburn, constipation, and bloating are common symptoms that appear when you begin intermittent fasting or any significant diet change. It happens because your digestive system is trying to adjust to the new eating patterns.

The gastric juice release in the digestive tract is regulated by the ghrelin hormone that causes the feeling of hunger. The body releases this hormone as per your eating schedules irrespective of the need for energy. It means that if regularly eat at 5 in the evening, the gut would release ghrelin at that time, even if you ate an hour ago. It would also lead to the release of gastric juices. When you don't eat anything, heartburn and bloating can occur.

However, you don't need to worry about it as these symptoms would also subside quickly. The ghrelin release would get adjusted to your new eating schedules within a few days.

Constipation can occur due to a change in your diet. Try to include more fiber-rich food in your diet, and the problem of constipation would also go away within a few days.

Dehydration

This can be a problem for women who are not very careful about drinking water. You must drink water whenever you feel thirsty. It is a misconception that you have to drink a specific quantity of water. Simply drink whenever you feel thirsty, and don't try to suppress your thirst.

You should also avoid overhydration as that will ultimately lead to loss of minerals through excessive urination.

Don't Overeat

This is a mistake women often make. Some women feel that because they will be having a long fasting period after the last meal, they overeat to avoid hunger pangs. This is a mistake. The last meal of the day should be moderate to light. This is the meal, after which your body will go into inactivity and hence the energy requirements would automatically go down.

If you overeat, your body will not get a chance to draw energy from the fat stores. Your last meal of the day should be light and fiber-rich.

Some women feel very hungry in the morning as they are coming out of the extended fasting period. They overeat, and that would also do no good to you. Overeating in the morning would make you feel lethargic and sleepy. The meal to break the fast should be nutrient-dense and balanced. However, it shouldn't be more in quantity.

Chapter 18: Goal Setting for Success and Motivation

The Key for Setting Milestones and Achieving Them

Goal Setting

It is very important to have specific goals when you begin any weight loss routine. Goals are empowering and help you muster the strength to keep moving toward them. There are only two big problems that people face while setting goals.

1. Very Big and Ambiguous Goals
2. Slow or No Progress

These are two common problems, and they will come in front when you don't plan things properly.

Very Big and Ambiguous Goals

It is always important to aim high and have big expectations but setting very big goals that aren't even clear in the definition may also lead to disappointments.

What I mean to say is that you want to get lean, and hence you set a goal that you want to lose weight and get very slim. This is a very vague definition, and you wouldn't have a way to measure your progress.

For instance, if you are suffering from morbid obesity or obesity, this goal is next to impossible in the near future. It would take a lot of time and effort. Another thing is the vague nature of the goal. You will have to set specific goals like you want to lose 10 pounds or 20 pounds in 6 months.

Having quantifiable goals is very helpful. You can always check your progress and have the aim in view. There is also a scope of relative improvement.

Slow or No Progress

This is a problem you would generally face when you don't break your goal into smaller milestones. You must always break your goals into smaller milestones so that at short intervals, you may have the feeling of accomplishment. This will keep you motivated.

For instance, if you have set a goal of losing 10 pounds in 2 months, you should break it into weekly milestones. It would come down to 1.25 pounds per week. The progress in the first few weeks may be slow, but you'll catch up later. Breaking down bigger goals into smaller milestones helps in keeping hold of the overall progress, and you also don't feel the progress stalled.

Ways to Remain Motivated

Weight loss can be a tiresome and backbreaking journey full of ups and downs. It is important that you keep yourself motivated and have your pillars of support, or else there are high chances of the resolve withering away.

Confide in Someone

You must have someone to talk to. It can be a friend of someone in your family who could provide you the required support in times of emotional lows.

Join Support Groups

Support groups are also very helpful as you can find people struggling with similar issues, and you can share your problems with them and learn from their experiences. Sharing problems is a good way to get over them easily.

Meditate

Meditation is also a good way to remain motivated. It helps you in keeping your mind calm and focused. Meditation also gives you a wider perspective of looking at the problem with a positive outlook.

Chapter 19: Maintaining The Desired Weight

Finally Breaking the Curse of Weight Relapse

Weight relapse is a big problem that women face very often, and it is also a cause of great disappointment. If not handled properly, weight relapse becomes a normal affair for people, and very often, women don't treat it as a sign of a bigger problem.

Weight relapse is a clear sign of a poor lifestyle. It should not happen. It signifies that the woman has poor control over her life.

Intermittent fasting is a great way to maintain any given weight and avoid weight relapses. It is simple to follow, and it prevents your weight issues from going out of hand.

There are 4 simple things that you must keep in mind if you want to avoid any kind of weight relapse.

1. Food
2. Exercise

3. Rest/Sleep
4. Healthy Routine

Food

We have already discussed food in detail in this book in the previous chapters. Food plays a very important role in your weight. Intermittent fasting helps you a lot as you don't have to bother any longer about the number of calories you are consuming. However, this doesn't mean that you can get reckless about your calorie intake. Food must be treated as a necessity, and overconsumption of food must be avoided. You should also avoid eating high-sugar foods and things made up of refined carbs.

Consuming a diet that lacks nutrients will make you feel hungry frequently, and maintaining the fasting hours will become a difficult task for you.

If you want to maintain a healthy weight, you must consume a nutrient-dense diet as per your caloric-requirement. Once in a while, in small quantities, you can also have the things you dearly want to eat, and that wouldn't have a big impact on your weight.

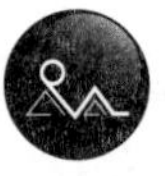
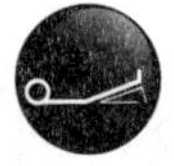

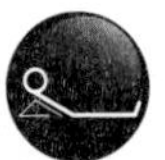

Exercise

Exercise is important for maintaining any specific weight. If you want to avoid weight relapse, you must exercise for a specific amount of time daily. Exercising in the morning is always the best, but if you can't find the time in the morning, you can even do it in the evening.

Even if you are not able to do rigorous high-intensity exercises, you must at least do light exercises. Leaving everything to intermittent fasting and food may not be a very good idea. The purpose of the intermittent fasting routine is to help you lead a healthy life.

Even light exercises can help you in not only burning some extra calories but also in building better immunity and tolerance. For instance, when you do any kind of exercise like running, swimming, or any other such exercise that puts a bit of stress on your body, the body starts releasing a chemical called nitric oxide, this chemical helps in making the blood vessels expand and contract better. Your blood vessels become more flexible. It gives your heart the right kind of exercise. This is very helpful in patients suffering from heart problems or high blood sugar as their blood vessels generally get very stiff and lose their ability to expand or contract properly. This is the cause of heart attacks.

Daily exercise, even in small amounts, can not only help you in maintaining your weight, but it would also help in keeping your healthy and safe.

Sleep

We have already discussed, sleep is very important when you are fasting. Your body is experiencing little positive stress, and sleeping can help the body in the repair and maintenance process. Inadequate sleep leads to higher stress in the body; It also causes insulin resistance in the body. People who usually work at night are more susceptible to weight gain. Your sleeping routine should be in accordance with your circadian rhythm.

Healthy Routine

This is a crucial thing that gets missed most of the time. If you want to maintain a healthy weight, you must maintain a healthy routine. Neither your mind should remain focused on food all the time, nor it should leave out daily exercise. A healthy routine would have a place for all the main ingredients.

Chapter 20: Meal Ideas

Low-Calorie Diet (1200 Calories)

Breakfast

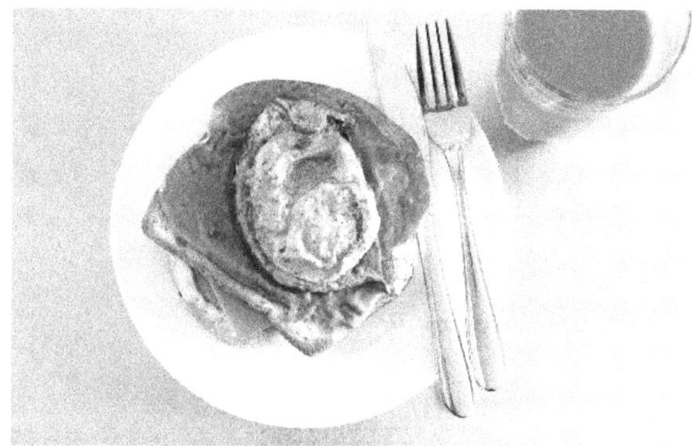

2 Poached Eggs

1 Orange

1 Slice of Avocado

Lunch

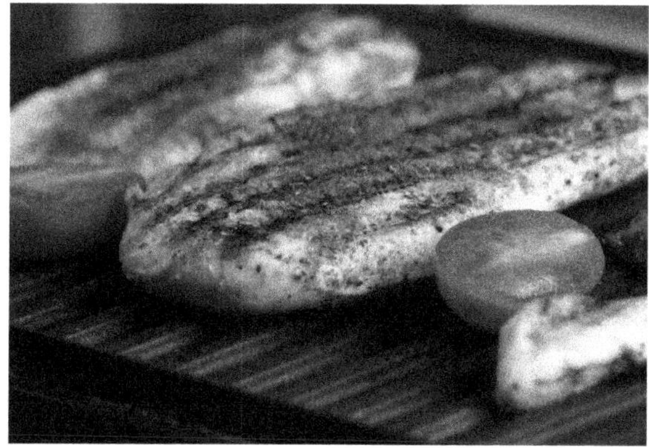

50g Grilled Chicken Breast

100ml Yogurt

Baked beans in tomato sauce

Cucumber and Lettuce salad garnished with olives

Ingredients for 4 persons

1/3 cup oil olive or vegetable oil

1/4 cup cider vinegar (or red wine vinegar)

2 tablespoons dijon mustard

3 tablespoons Worcestershire sauce

2 tablespoons lemon juice

1 tablespoon salt

1 tablespoon pepper

2 tablespoons Italian seasoning

1 teaspoon garlic powder

1 tablespoon sugar

4 boneless skinless chicken breasts

Instructions

Combine all ingredients in a bowl or freezer bag. Add chicken and toss well to combine.

Marinade for a 30 minutes (or up to 4 hours) before cooking chicken.

Preheat grill to medium high heat.

Place chicken on the grill for 7-8 minutes. Flip over and cook an additional 7-8 minutes or until no pink remains and chicken reaches 165°F.

Rest 3-5 minutes before slicing.

Baked beans in tomato sauce

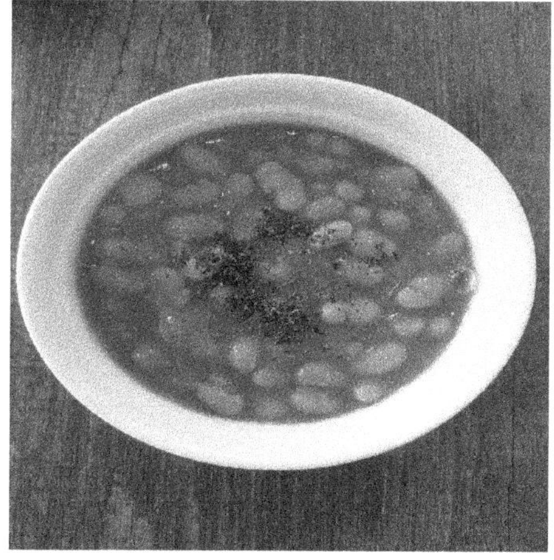

If you want to save time, you can used canned beans instead of dry. Use 3 or 4 15-ounce cans, drained and rinsed and proceed to step 3. If you want a vegetarian version, skip the bacon, increase the olive oil, and use vegetable stock.

INGREDIENTS

1 pound dry cannellini, borlotti or Great Northern beans

1 tablespoon extra virgin olive oil

1/4 pound bacon or pancetta, roughly chopped

1/2 medium onion, chopped

4 garlic cloves, chopped

1 tablespoon fresh sage, minced (can sub fresh rosemary)

1/2 to 1 teaspoon chile flakes (depending on how spicy you want it)

2 tablespoons honey

1/4 cup tomato paste

1 15-ounce can crushed tomatoes or tomato sauce

2 cups beef or chicken stock (use gluten-free stock for gluten-free version)

Salt

1/2 cup chopped fresh parsley

2 tablespoons balsamic vinegar

Instructions

1 Soak the beans in water: Pre-soak the beans, either by covering with two inches of water and soaking overnight, or by pouring boiling water over them and soaking them for an hour.

2 Drain beans, cover with water, cook until tender: Drain the beans and put them in a medium-sized pot and cover with 2 inches of water. Bring to a simmer, cover, reduce the heat to a low simmer and cook until the beans are just soft enough to eat, about 1 hour, give or take 15 minutes or so, depending on how old the beans are (older beans will take longer to cook).

3 Cook bacon or pancetta: Preheat the oven to 325°F. In a 3 or 4 quart heavy-bottomed, oven-proof, lidded pot such as a Dutch oven, heat the olive oil over medium heat. Add the bacon or pancetta and cook slowly until lightly browned and crispy.

4 Sauté onions: Add the chopped onions and increase the heat to medium-high. Cook, stirring often, until the onions begin to brown. Use a wooden spoon to scrape any browned bits off the bottom of the pot.

5 Add garlic, chili flakes, sage, then add tomatoes and stock: Add the garlic, chile flakes and sage and cook for 1-2 minutes, then add the honey and tomato paste. Stir well to combine.

Add the tomatoes or tomato sauce and the stock. Bring to a simmer. Taste for salt and add some if needed.

6 Add the beans, cover, cook in oven: Drain the beans and add them to the pot. Stir well.

Cover the pot and cook in a 325°F oven for 1 hour and 15 minutes.

If still a bit wet, remove the cover and cook for 15 minutes more.

Note that the cooking time will depend on several things, the most important being how thoroughly the beans were cooked to begin with when they were simmered.

If the beans are still a bit hard when they go in the oven, it may take several hours to soften them, once the tomato and honey have been added.

7 Stir in parsley and balsamic vinegar: Right before serving, gently stir in the chopped parsley and balsamic vinegar. Taste for salt, add more if needed to taste.

Serve either hot or at room temperature.

Dinner

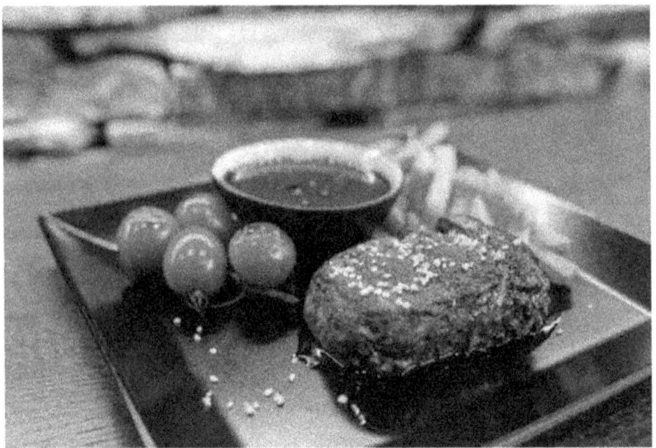

50g steak pan-fried with half a cup of cooked lentils

150g Sliced Peaches.

Ingredients for 4 persons

250g lentils

200g rainbow or swiss chard

100g kale

3-4 tbsp extra-virgin oil, plus extra for drizzling

2 garlic cloves

Handful spring onions

2-3 tbsp red wine vinegar

4 British steaks (sirloin or rump)

½-1 lemon

Cook the lentils for 15-20 minutes in a large pan of salted boiling water until just tender. Meanwhile, separate the chard stems and leaves; chop the stems into 2cm slices and tear the leaves into quarters.

Heat a frying pan with a glug of olive oil, add the chard and kale, then season. Cook over a high heat, tossing, for 2-3 minutes until wilted and tender. Transfer to a large bowl. Drain the cooked lentils, then add to the bowl with 3-4 tbsp olive oil and season. Crush the garlic, slice the spring onions and toss with the lentils and vinegar to taste.

Wipe the frying pan clean and put back over a high heat. Brush the steaks with oil and season. Fry for 11/2 minutes on each side for rare; 2 minutes for medium-rare; 3 minutes for medium-well done. Rest the steaks for 2-3 minutes.

Tip any resting juices into the lentils and squeeze in lemon juice to taste. Toss, then serve with the steaks.

Medium Calorie Diet (1500 Calories)

Breakfast

Breakfast Sausage

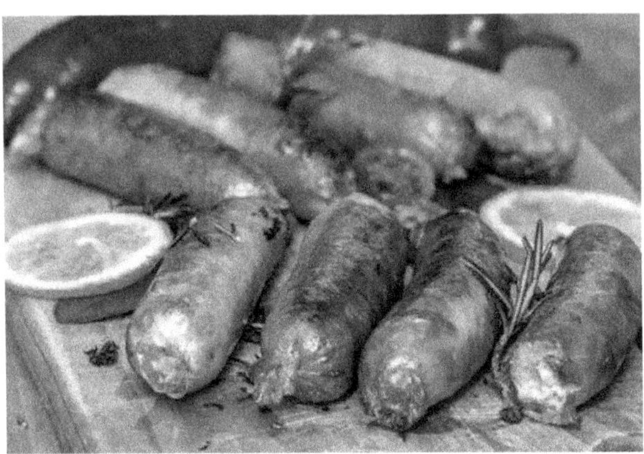

Ingredients

10 pounds boneless pork butt/shoulder(this cut is recommended for the right ratio of lean meat to fat)

3/4 cup chopped fresh sage

3 tablespoons chopped fresh thyme

5 tablespoons sea salt

2 tablespoons ground ginger

1 1/2 tablespoons freshly ground white pepper

1 1/2 tablespoons freshly ground black pepper

2 tablespoons minced fresh garlic

1 tablespoons ground nutmeg

2 cups ice water

Natural sheep casings (3/4 inch/20 mm, about 30 feet), soaked and thoroughly rinsed

For a sweeter variation: Add 1 cup of maple syrup along with the ice water

Instructions

Cut the pork into 1/2 inch chunks and freeze them for about 45 minutes to get them to a temperature of 32 degrees F (0 celsius). Grind the pork through a 1/4 inch (6mm) die (I use this meat grinder). Grind the meat quickly into the bowl of a stand mixer (ideally have the bowl set atop an ice bath to keep the meat cold) and then grind it all a second time. Chill the meat in the refrigerator while you assemble the spice mixture.

In a bowl combine the salt, sage, thyme, ginger, white and black pepper, garlic and nutmeg.

Remove the ground meat from the fridge and place it on the stand mixer fitted with a paddle attachment. (If you have room in your freezer, pre-chill the mixing bowl.) Add the spice mixture and the ice water. Mix it with the paddle for 3-4 minutes until threads begin to appear in the meat (if you take a clump of meat and pull it apart with your fingers you will see tiny threads pulling apart). Chill the mixture in the fridge while you prepare the sausage stuffer. Take a bit of the meat mixture, fry it up, taste it and adjust the seasonings if needed.

Thread the sausage stuffer with the prepared sheep casings, fill the sausage stuffer with the meat mixture, and fill the casings being careful to avoid air gaps while also not overstuffing the casings. Twist the sausages into links. Use a sausage pricker to prick any air bubbles out of the links.

Cook the sausages by heating up some oil in a frying pan and frying the sausages on each side for about 3 minutes until browned and done in the middle (internal temperature of 155 degrees F).

OR you can poach the sausages (do not boil) in lightly salted water until their internal temperature reaches 155 degrees F, then let them cool in ice water, wrap them and store in the fridge for up to a week or in the freezer for up to 2 months.

Notes

It is essential to keep the meat sufficiently cold throughout the process so that proper definition between the lean meat and fat is visible, otherwise if the fat is mashed and smeared in the meat the sausages won't have a good texture (if this happens use the ground sausage for cooking as you would ground Italian sausage). Keeping the meat properly chilled will also prevent bacteria growth.

If you prefer, you can skip the sausage-stuffing process and simply form the mixture into patties and fry them. (Feel free to half or quarter the recipe if not making it in bulk.)

Calories: 103kcal | Protein: 14g | Fat: 4g | Saturated Fat: 1g.

Lunch

Casserole of Chicken and Mushroom 100g served with a cup of cooked rice and half a cup of cooked peas and beetroot salad.

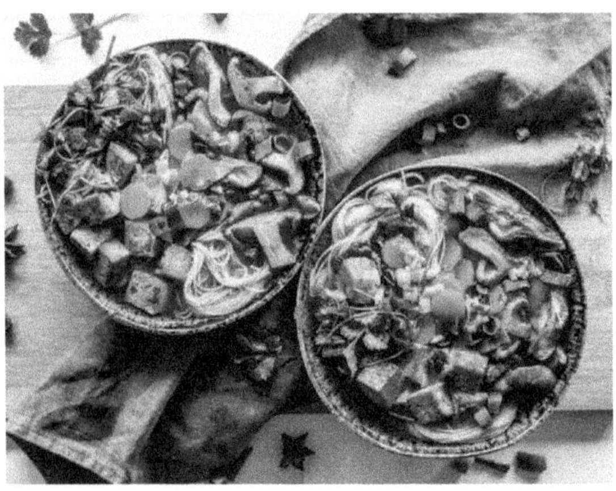

Ingredients

5 chicken breasts chopped into big chunks or strips

9 tbsp plain/all purpose flour all purpose flour

1 tsp salt

1 tsp black pepper

2 tbsp vegetable oil

2 tbsp unsalted butter

3 brown onions peeled and finely diced

5 cloves garlic peeled and minced

1 tsp dried thyme

½ tsp celery salt optional

1 litre chicken stock

300 ml milk

2 tbsp freshly squeezed lemon juice

16-20 chestnut mushrooms thickly sliced (white mushrooms or baby portabella are good too)

240 ml double (heavy) cream

Optional: 3tbsp cornflour/cornstarch mixed with 5 tbsp cold water – to make a slurry

Small bunch parsley chopped

Serve with:

Mashed potato

Sprouts

Peas

Sweetcorn

Instructions

Place the chicken in a bowl with 6 tablespoons of the flour plus 1/2 tsp each of salt and pepper. Toss to cover the chicken in the flour and seasoning.

Heat the oil over a high heat in a large frying pan (skillet) and add the chicken. Brown all over (it doesn't need to be cooked through at this point). Remove from the pan with a slotted spoon and put to one side.

Place the butter in the same frying pan and melt over a low-medium heat. Add the onions, garlic, thyme and celery salt and cook for 5 minutes until the onion softens. Sprinkle on the remaining 3 tbsp of flour and stir for a minute (it will be lumpy).

Pour in a splash of the stock and stir, using a whisk until combined. Continue to add in stock, a little at a time, whilst stirring, until all the stock is added and you have a smooth sauce with no lumps (the onions will still be in there though - so it will look a little lumpy because of that).

Add the milk and continue to stir over the heat until the sauce thickens, then add in the lemon juice.

Add the mushrooms, the chicken and the remaining 1/2 tsp of salt and pepper. Place a lid on the pan and simmer gently on the hob for 20 minutes.

Alternatively you can transfer to a casserole dish at this point. Cover with foil and place in the oven at 175C/350F for 30 minutes

Remove the lid and stir in the cream, then heat through for a further 5 minutes (place back in the oven if oven cooking).

Remove the lid and test for seasoning. Add a little more salt and pepper if needed.

If you'd like the sauce to be any thicker, then at this point you can stir in the cornflour slurry. Add a little splash at a time, whilst stirring, until you get the thickness you want.

Serve the casserole with a cup of cooked rice, beet salad and a sprinkling of parsley.

Dinner

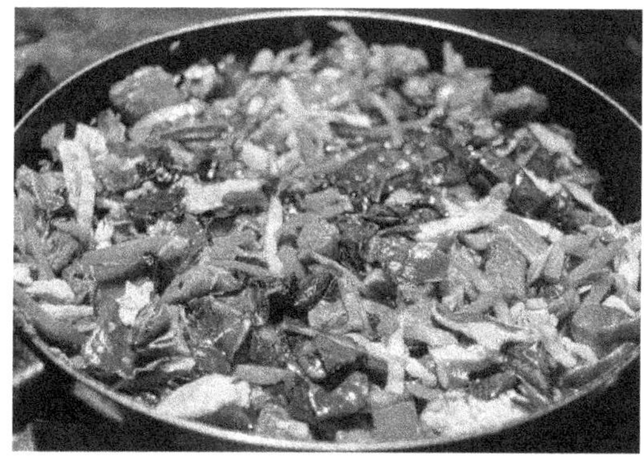

100g pan-fried salmon with a cup of cooked brown rice

Half cup cooked tomatoes and onions with lettuce and sliced oranges on the top. You can also add mayo sauce for taste

50g yogurt

High-Calorie Diet (1800 Calories)

Breakfast

Whole Grain Southwestern Toast

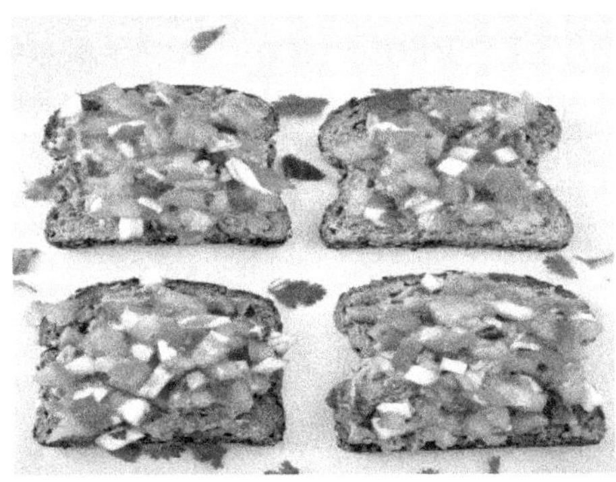

Ingredients

3 tomatoes, diced

1/2 cup diced red onion

1 T chopped cilantro

1 clove garlic, minced

Juice from 1 lime

Sea salt to taste

2 large avocadoes, mashed

4 slices eureka! Sweet Baby Grains

Instructions

Mix all ingredients, except the avocado and bread, in a bowl.

Toast the bread.

Spread some pureed avocado onto each slice of toast.

Add the salsa mixture on top of each slice.

Serve immediately for best results. Enjoy!

Lunch

Chicken Teriyaki Meatball Bowls

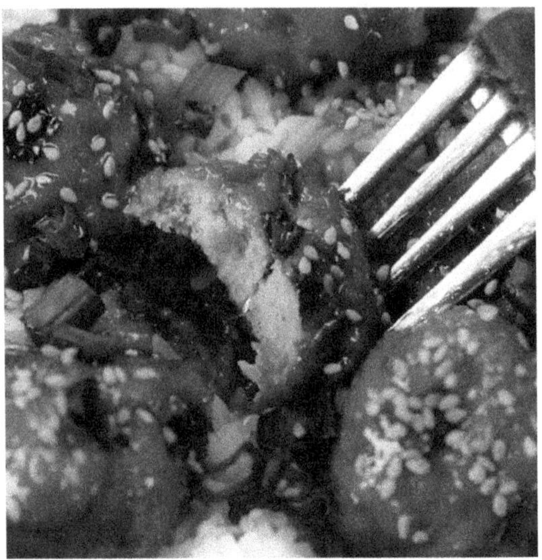

Ingredients

for 3 servings

MEATBALLS

1 lb ground chicken (455 g)

1 egg

1 cup panko breadcrumbs (50 g)

1 teaspoon garlic, minced

2 teaspoons fresh ginger, shredded

1 tablespoon soy sauce

2 tablespoons scallion, chopped

½ teaspoon salt

¼ teaspoon pepper

GLAZE

½ cup soy sauce (120 mL)

½ tablespoon sesame oil

1 tablespoon rice vinegar

2 tablespoons honey

½ tablespoon sriracha

½ cup brown sugar (110 g)

2 teaspoons garlic, minced

2 teaspoons fresh ginger, shredded

CORNSTARCH SLURRY

½ tablespoon cornstarch

½ tablespoon water

GARNISH

sesame seed, optional

scallion, optional

Preparation

Preheat the oven to 400ºF (200ºC). Line a baking sheet with parchment paper and set aside.

Combine all ingredients for the meatballs in a bowl.

Mix until all ingredients are well-blended.

Use an ice cream scoop or a spoon and form into meatballs. Place on the baking sheet.

Bake for 20-25 minutes (until lightly browned and the chicken is cooked through).

In the meantime, prepare the glaze! Pour soy sauce, rice vinegar, sesame oil, honey, sriracha, garlic, ginger, and brown sugar into a sauce pan.

Turn on medium heat, and stir until the sugar has dissolved.

Then, pour in the cornstarch slurry and whisk until the sauce has thickened (about 5 minutes).

Add the meatballs to the sauce pan and evenly coat them with the teriyaki glaze.

Serve over rice or serve on their own! Garnish with Scallions and Sesame Seeds.

Enjoy!

Dinner

Shrimp and Vegetable Skillet with Sausage

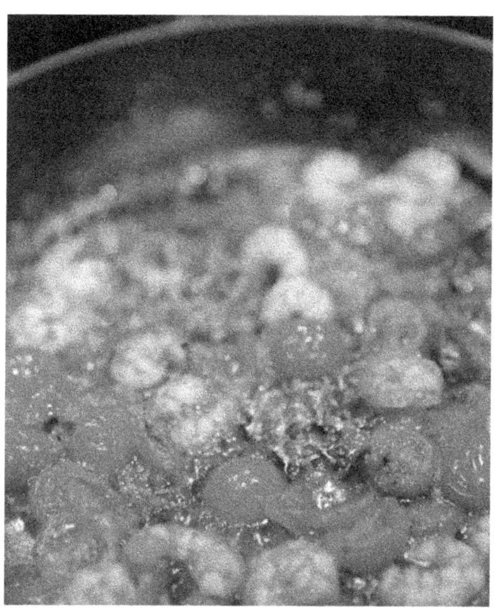

HOW TO MAKE SHRIMP AND VEGETABLES:

1. Cut the vegetables into bite-sized pieces.

2. Place the shrimp into a medium bowl and add the Cajun seasoning, paprika, salt, and olive oil. Mix well.

3. Heat a large skillet over medium-high heat. Add the shrimp and cook for about 6-7 minutes, or until cooked through. Remove the shrimp from the skillet and set aside.

4. To the same skillet, add the garlic, butter, and vegetables. Season with salt, and stir-fry for about 10 minutes, or until the vegetables are tender.

5. Return the shrimp to the skillet, stir well, and garnish with parsley. Serve.

WHAT TO SERVE SHRIMP AND VEGETABLES WITH

This tasty dish could be served as is, with some crusty bread on the side. It will also pair well with cooked rice, quinoa, couscous, and pasta.

This Shrimp and Vegetable Skillet stays well in the refrigerator and tastes great the next day. It also makes a wonderful meal prep option. Enjoy!

Conclusion

Thank you for making it through to the end of this book, let's hope it was informative and able to provide you with all of the tools you need to achieve your goals whatever they may be.

Intermittent fasting has emerged as a great way to lose body fat and gain good health. Yet, many women fail to get all the benefits of this wonderful process due to a lack of knowledge of the process. This book has tried to bring all the important points on the forefront so that you can get all the benefits of intermittent fasting without having to face the negative effects.

All you need to do is follow the information given in the book and stick to the adopted routine.

You can also get all the benefits of the process by following the simple steps given in the book.

I hope that this book is really able to help you in achieving your goals.

APPENDIX

Cooking Conversion Charts

Volume (liquid)	
US Customary	Metric
1/8 teaspoon	.6 ml
1/4 teaspoon	1.2 ml
1/2 teaspoon	2.5 ml
3/4 teaspoon	3.7 ml
1 teaspoon	5 ml
1 tablespoon	15 ml
2 tablespoon or 1 fluid ounce	30 ml
1/4 cup or 2 fluid ounces	59 ml
1/3 cup	79 ml
1/2 cup	118 ml
2/3 cup	158 ml
3/4 cup	177 ml
1 cup or 8 fluid ounces	237 ml
2 cups or 1 pint	473 ml
4 cups or 1 quart	946 ml
8 cups or 1/2 gallon	1.9 liters
1 gallon	3.8 liters

Weight (mass)	
US contemporary (ounces)	Metric (grams)
1/2 ounce	14 grams
1 ounce	28 grams
3 ounces	85 grams
3.53 ounces	100 grams
4 ounces	113 grams
8 ounces	227 grams
12 ounces	340 grams
16 ounces or 1 pound	454 grams

Oven Temperatures	
US contemporary	Metric
250° F	121° C
300° F	149° C
350° F	177° C
400° F	204° C
450° F	232° C

Volume Equivalents (liquid)		
3 teaspoons	1 tablespoon	0.5 fluid ounce
2 tablespoons	1/8 cup	1 fluid ounce
4 tablespoons	1/4 cup	2 fluid ounces
5 1/3 tablespoons	1/3 cup	2.7 fluid ounces
8 tablespoons	1/2 cup	4 fluid ounces
12 tablespoons	3/4 cup	6 fluid ounces
16 tablespoons	1 cup	8 fluid ounces
2 cups	1 pint	16 fluid ounces
2 pints	1 quart	32 fluid ounces
4 quarts	1 gallon	128 fluid ounces

The Others Books By Maybelle Campbell

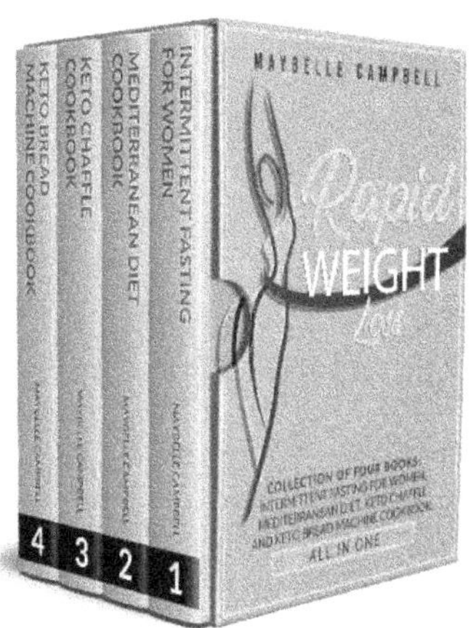

RAPID WEIGHT LOSS

Collection of Four Books: Intermittent Fasting for Women, Mediterranean Diet, Keto Chaffle and Keto Bread Machine Cookbook

(All in One).

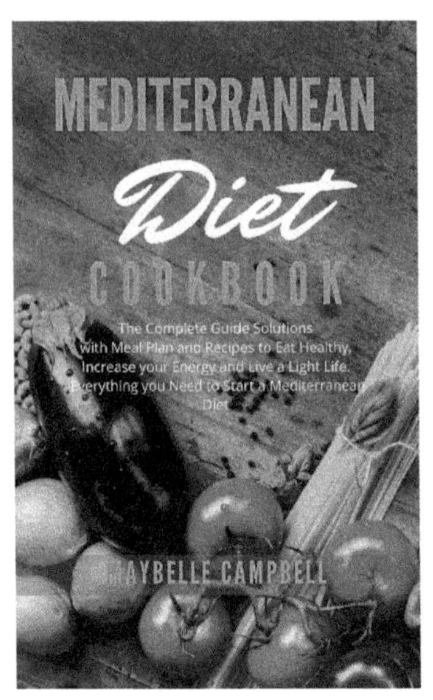

MEDITERRANEAN DIET COOKBOOK

The Complete Guide Solutions with Meal Plan and Recipes to Eat Healthy, Increase your Energy and Live a Light Life. Everything you Need to Start a Mediterranean Diet

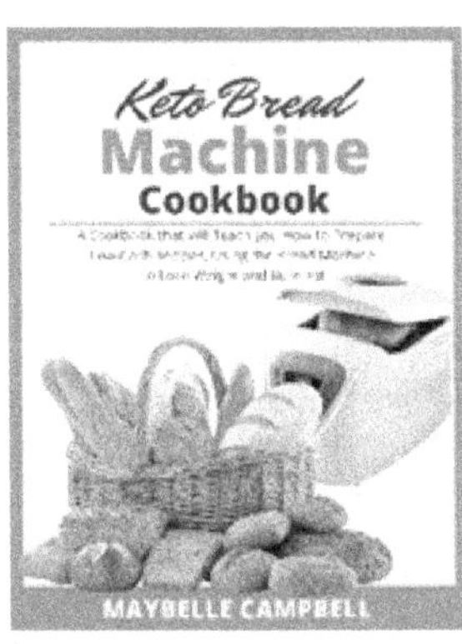

KETO BREAD MACHINE COOKBOOK

A Cookbook that will Teach you How to Prepare Low-Carb Recipes, Using the Bread Machine to Lose Weight and Burn Fat

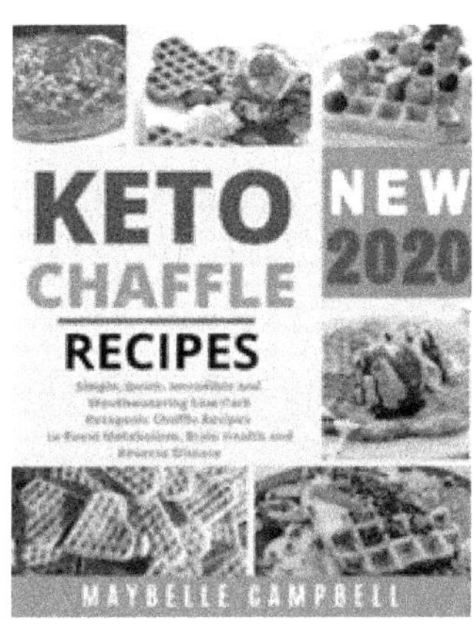

KETO CHAFFLE RECIPES

Simple, Quick, Incredible and Mouthwatering Low-Carb Ketogenic Chaffle Recipes to Boost Metabolism, Brain Health and Reverse Disease

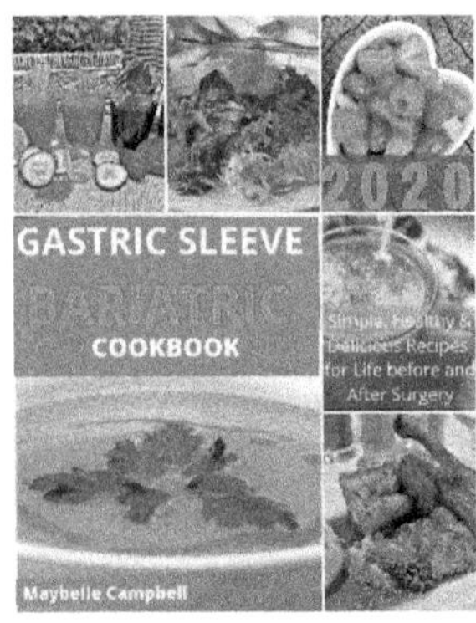

GASTRIC SLEEVE BARIATRIC COOKBOOK

Simple, Healthy & Delicious Recipes for Life before and After Surgery

CPSIA information can be obtained
at www.ICGtesting.com
Printed in the USA
BVHW040852251120
594183BV00017B/426